AUTOIMMUNE

THE CAUSE AND THE CURE

AUTOIMMUNE

THE CAUSE AND THE CURE

By Annesse Brockley and Kristin Urdiales

For additional information, please visit: www.NatureHadItFirst.com

Copyright © 2011, 2012
First Edition September 2011
Second Edition May 2012

All rights reserved. No part of this book may be reproduced or transmitted in any form without permission in writing from the authors.

ISBN: 978-0-9836037-0-2

A MESSAGE TO THE READER

Neither the publisher, nor the authors are engaged in rendering professional advice or services to the reader. This book is not intended as a substitute for medical advice from a licensed health care practitioner. Any decision involving the treatment of an illness should be made only after consulting a physician. Do not adjust your medication in any way without professional medical advice. The reader should consult his or her medical, health, or other competent professional before adopting any of the suggestions in this book or drawing inferences from it. The authors and publisher specifically disclaim all responsibility for any liability, loss, or risk, personal or otherwise, which is incurred as a consequence, directly or indirectly, of the use and application of any of the contents of this book.

ACKNOWLEDGEMENTS

This book is dedicated to the many sufferers of autoimmune disease.

To Sally Fallon and Rosemary Gladstar – thank you for laying the foundation that others can now build upon.

Becky Pullen, Denise Dunckley, and Nancy Arey – we owe you a sincere debt of gratitude for your scientific research and tireless efforts.

To our family and friends – thank you for your love and support.

Above all, we thank The God of All Comfort.

FROM THE AUTHORS

This book has brought together scientific research from around the world, which we believe uncovers the cause of autoimmune disease. This collective evidence offers valid proof, not only of the cause of autoimmune disease, but also of the only possible way to cure it.

Every symptom of autoimmune disease can now be clearly explained and traced back to its origin. The evidence proves that these diseases share a common source, and that this source is not viral, bacterial, or genetic, but originates with a fundamental lack of nutrients that are essential to the functioning of your body.

What began as a personal journey of pain and suffering, has resulted in life-saving knowledge for autoimmune sufferers everywhere.

-Annesse Brockley and Kristin Urdiales

Autoimmune: The Cause and Cure
by Annesse Brockley and Kristin Urdiales

Copyright © 2011, 2012 Nature Had It First, LLC

No part of this book may be reproduced in any form; written, electronic, recording, or photocopying without the written permission of the publisher or author.
The exception would be in the case of brief quotations embodied in the critical articles or reviews and pages where permission is specifically granted by the publisher or author.

Although every precaution has been taken to verify the accuracy of the information contained herein, the author and publisher assume no responsibility for any errors or omissions. No liability is assumed for damages that may result from the use of information contained within.

Published by Nature Had It First, LLC
195 Pine Cone Ave
Spearfish, SD 57783

ISBN: 978-0-9836037-0-2

Health

First Edition September 2011
Second Edition May 2012
Printed in the United States of America

Website: www.NatureHadItFirst.com

Cover and Interior Design: Epicenter Creative

CONTENTS

The book is divided into three chapters:
The Story, The Discovery, and The Recovery

CHAPTER 1 THE STORY-ANNESSE'S STORY 1

CHAPTER 2 THE DISCOVERY
DNase 1 10
Pancreatic Enzymes, Vitamin B12 and Proteins 16
Homocysteine 69
Tumor Necrosis Factor (TNF): Its Role in Autoimmune Disease 115
Signs and Symptoms of Pancreatic Enzyme Deficiency Disease 123
The FM Differential Diagnosis List – Don't Miss This One 137
Summarizing the Emerging Theory About the Origins of Autoimmunity 148

CHAPTER 3 THE RECOVERY
Food as Medicine 150
Healing Your Gut 157
Things That Destroy Beneficial Gut Flora 159
A Processed-Food Future 174
Proteins 176
Beverages 183
Non-Organic Foods 192
Personal Care Products and Indoor Air Pollution 196
Yeast and Gluten 197
The Foods That Will Bring You Back "The Fermented Foods Diet" 200

QUESTION AND ANSWERS 227
RESOURCES 231
REFERENCES 233

Chapter 1 THE STORY

I awoke that summer morning in 1992 excited about the coming day and evening. I would be attending my 20-year high school reunion. I was looking forward to catching up with my old classmates and reliving a time of life that, although I didn't miss, was filled with good memories. The reunion did not disappoint and I was sorry to see it end. I also had the added surprise of being given the title of 'best figure' by my classmates. Instead of acknowledging the classmates who had become brain surgeons or political leaders, I guess we figured that after 20 years, the only accomplishment that really mattered was whether or not we had gained weight. When I arrived home that evening, I was not just tired, I was exhausted. Unfortunately, that feeling of exhaustion would be the beginning of a new and very different chapter in my life.

Being tired was nothing new. I had pushed myself daily for years to run the business that my husband and I had started, and to raise a teenage daughter and a five-year-old son. I had always been active and I loved to exercise. I regularly rode my bike down a nearby canyon and walked virtually everywhere. On our way home from somewhere, I would often shout out, "Stop the car!" I would then jump out and walk the rest of the way. Even though I exercised, it was not as if I was filled with energy. I was often tired, but I pushed myself thinking that it was the right thing to do. I thought exercise would give me energy. In a healthy person, that's true. However, as I learned years later, energy is what your body makes to allow you to exercise and lead a busy life. If you don't give your body the nutrients it needs to create energy, you will someday cross the line from tired to exhausted. That is what happened to me that eventful summer day. My body crossed the line, and it would be a long time before I was able to find my way back.

New and disturbing symptoms were soon added to the overwhelming exhaustion. I had gone to Denver for a few days of vacation with my husband. One morning, after having a latte and croissant at a French bistro close to our hotel, we walked to Washington Park to get some exercise. It was a ritual I loved; exercise and food together. As we began our walk, I could feel my legs start to tighten and then completely cramp up to the point of total immobility. After some time, I was able to limp my way back to our car. I was confused and a little scared, but I thought, or hoped, it was something that would pass. It did not.

The muscle pain and inflammation that began that day were now part of my new and increasingly terrifying life. New symptoms were added soon afterwards. I noticed that my nose would start running whenever I ate something. I also started having daily migraines. They were like no headaches I had ever experienced and anything could trigger them. Just bending over to pick something off the floor could trigger a headache that would last for days. By now, I was also constantly running a low-grade fever. The symptoms were very flu-like. I was achy and feverish. It was time to go see a doctor.

My blood work from the doctor's visit came back showing a high sedimentation rate and elevated potassium. Apparently, the high potassium levels are indicative of someone that has been injured in some way. The doctor kept asking me if I had fallen or had suffered some muscle trauma. "No, nothing," I said. The doctor prescribed an antibiotic. What for, I wasn't sure. I started to take it, knowing it was not going to fix what was wrong with me. By the fourth day, I began to feel worse and stopped taking it.

The next few years went by in a blur of pain. I was spending most of my day in bed. At times, I was unable to wash my hair or even climb a flight of stairs. My chest hurt when I would take a breath, and at times it felt as though someone was driving a nail through my foot. I could sit at the computer for short periods of time, but would have to support my elbow with my other arm while I moved the mouse. I would pay dearly for that brief indiscretion with increased pain and fatigue. I also had nosebleeds all the time that I couldn't stop. I knew I was dying and needed to find answers.

One day, a friend suggested I get tested for food allergies. Although food intolerances are more common, true food allergies occur in 1 in 25 adults, and recent studies indicate their incidence is on the rise (National Institutes of Health, 2010). Apparently, a food allergy can be identified by an assay that uses a small amount of blood to check for antibodies against specific foods. I traveled to a Denver hospital for the testing. They tested me for 25 different foods on the first panel. I went home to wait for the results. When they called with the results, my husband happened to answer the phone. I was glad he did. This was the first time I had proof that something was seriously wrong with me. They said, "We have never seen anything like this, your wife is highly allergic to everything we tested her for."

The list included brown rice, green tea, broccoli, dairy, eggs, wheat, you name it—everything! I took the list they sent of the different foods to the local health food store, thinking that if I just didn't eat those things, I would get well. I would've done anything to get better. As I walked around the store, picking up different foods and reading the labels, I realized there wasn't one thing I could eat. I left the store in tears. I made a decision that day to just do the best I could. I would try to eat as healthy as possible.

Previously, I had never given much thought to my diet. I wasn't overweight and I ate what most other people did. We dined out at restaurants a lot because of our busy schedules, and being in a small town, there weren't many dining options. Almost daily, before I got sick, my husband and I would meet somewhere for lunch. It was usually the first thing I would eat that day. Most often, being a creature of habit, I would have a grilled ham and cheese sandwich with some fries and a few cups of coffee. Dinner was usually something similar. I remember thinking one day that I hadn't eaten a fruit or vegetable for almost three weeks. "That can't be good," I thought. Turns out, I was right.

My new diet progressed slowly, but steadily over the next few years. My teenage daughter was a ready and willing participant in this endeavor. She had begun to experience frequent headaches and after seeing what had happened to me, she was going to avoid the same fate if she could. One of my most vivid memories is of the night we both sat at our dining room table staring reluctantly at the salad before us. The idea of eating it with a fork just made it more disagreeable, so we picked up each leaf individually with our fingers. We weren't trying to enjoy it; we were just trying to get it down.

During the same time I was trying to change my diet, I had remembered a friend that was suffering with a debilitating stomach problem. She tried everything she could to obtain relief, including traveling to a Chinese herbalist in Los Angeles. The herbalist gave her a tea that included worms! I couldn't imagine how anyone could be so desperate that they would drink something with worms in it. Since she got better, it wasn't long before even I was willing to try worm tea if it would help.

So, my husband and I took a trip to Los Angeles. As we walked into the small cramped shop in Chinatown, we were greeted by a vast array of very strange sights and smells. There were seahorses in jars and creatures I had never seen before. The shelves were lined with herbs, dried roots, and flowers. It smelled musty and pungent. I was told to wait in a small back room. Before long, we were escorted into an even smaller, dimmer room with a curtain across the doorway. The Chinese doctor sat behind a desk and my husband and I sat down on a small couch. He did not speak English, and I didn't speak Chinese, so we just looked at each other. Before long, he just said, "lupus."

I turned to my husband and said, "What did he say?"

"I think he said lupus," my husband responded.

The Chinese doctor nodded and began to write on a pad. He handed me 'the prescription' to be filled out at the counter in front. I was just going to go with it. I didn't think I had anything to lose. As I handed the Chinese woman at the counter my prescription, I said, "No bugs!"

"Oh, you vegetarian?" she asked.

"Yes," I lied, with no remorse to this day.

I returned home with renewed hope. I was to make the herbs he had given me into a tea and drink about four cups a day. The tea was the most awful tasting and smelling concoction I had ever experienced. When I took a drink, I would shove a lemon wedge in my mouth to take the taste away and to keep myself from throwing up. It made my house smell as bad as the tea tasted. I did start to feel slightly better though, so I kept drinking it. Once a week, a new packet of herbs would arrive in the mail, and I would diligently force myself to make the tea and drink it.

My first indication that something was not quite right with the tea was on a short trip I had taken. If I went anywhere, I would take my Chinese cooking pot and a small hot plate to cook the herbs in the hotel room. I still can't believe someone didn't report me for doing something, if not illegal, just plain weird. One day, while cooking the herbs, I walked into the bathroom to check on them. A big cockroach looking thing was trying to escape from the boiling water! I tried to smash it with the lid and was horrified that it had come from the herbs I had been drinking.

Back home a week later, I opened up a newly delivered package of herbs to prepare my tea. I took one look and started screaming uncontrollably. My husband came running from his office. There were, what I thought to be, numerous spiders scattered throughout my herbs. I could barely speak, but I managed to point and say, "Spiders!"

"Calm down, calm down," he said in the most soothing tone he could muster. "They are not spiders."

I took a deep breath and started to relax, "They are beetles," he explained.

I couldn't believe I had been drinking beetles! I picked up the herbs and headed toward the back door. We were having a snowstorm, but I opened the door and threw them outside.

"What are you doing? That's $100 worth of herbs," my husband protested.

I turned to him and said, "We have herbs in this country and I'm going to learn about them."

I knew deep down that the food allergies I had were just a symptom of an unidentified disease. I decided to go back to Denver for some additional testing. From different things I had read, and from the symptoms I had, I was afraid I might have something like scleroderma. The results were given to me at the doctor's office a few days later.

"We think you have lupus," he said, "but we need to see if you develop any more symptoms. For now, we're diagnosing you with chronic fatigue syndrome and fibromyalgia." I was relieved to have some idea of what was going on.

Not long after, my husband and I took a short summer excursion to Aspen, Colorado. I would spend most of the time in the hotel room, but was able to take a short walk during the day. My husband would go out to dinner alone and bring back something for me. It was the best I could do and I was just grateful to be there. That time in Aspen, being exposed to the high-altitude sun, ushered in the symptom that would eventually lead me to the cure for my sickness. I looked in the mirror one evening, after I had spent a few hours outside, and noticed that my face, which up until now had a very faint, rosy color across the bridge of my nose and cheeks, was now becoming more red and rash-like. Day by day, it continued to worsen. I now realize that the Chinese doctor had seen the beginnings of that rash and that is how he knew I had lupus. All my other symptoms intensified as well. It felt like I had a bad flu that would not go away.

After returning home, I made an appointment to see a dermatologist. Just sitting in his office, even with people used to seeing rashes and skin diseases, I was getting many stares. The rash was inflamed and bright red. I was taken to an examining room and when the doctor entered the room, he took one look at me and exclaimed, "You have lupus!"

This was the third time I had heard that diagnosis. I was so sick by now that it didn't really matter to me what the name of the disease was. The rash that had appeared on my face would be with me daily for the next ten years.

It was so noticeable that it made being in public very difficult emotionally. Once, while in a mall with my daughter, she wanted to stop by the makeup counter at Neiman Marcus. I said, "No way am I going in there!" The bright fluorescent lights made my rash look even worse. She assured me no one would say anything to me. I told her I would wait by the entrance. I stood there uncomfortably while she approached the makeup counter.

Then, from about twenty feet away, one of the makeup personnel yelled, "Excuse me, excuse me! Did you just have laser surgery done?"

"No," I said, "I have lupus."

"We have something for that!" she hollered back.

I was mortified. I couldn't get out of there fast enough.

My health continued on a downhill slide. It got to where it was too painful to travel by car, so we purchased a van with a bed in it to take necessary trips. I was getting worse and I was desperate to find answers.

Because of my beetle juice experience, I decided to take my herbal treatment into my own hands. I began by reading every book on alternative treatments that I could find. When in Denver, one of the activities that filled my time was going to a wonderful bookstore called, 'The Tattered Cover.' My husband would drop me off, and I would head to the herbal section, find a book I had not read, and sit in one of their oversized chairs for hours. I would purchase the books I wanted and have a supply of reading material for several months after I returned home. One day, I entered the store and found my way to the health and herbal section. As I looked up at the hundreds of books on the shelves, I realized I could not find one that I had not read. Now what, I thought? I decided to contact the authors of the books that I had found most helpful. I did this by phone and sometimes by traveling to their hometowns. On one of these trips, we chartered a small plane to fly us to Santa Fe, New Mexico, to visit Daniel Gagnon. He is well known for making a line of herbal products that I found helpful. The unpressurized airplane made me so ill that we had to find a landing site virtually in the middle of nowhere. When we finally arrived in Santa Fe and made it to the hotel room, I was too exhausted to attend the appointment I had made with Daniel. I didn't even have enough strength to lift the receiver to call him.

I continued to learn and research until I was comfortable that I had learned all that I possibly could on the subject of herbal treatments for lupus. I felt that my herbs and diet would keep me alive long enough to find out why I was so sick. I took no pharmaceuticals during this time, whatsoever. Not even an aspirin. I didn't want to mask the symptoms, as I felt they would eventually lead me to the cause.

My continued research led me to contact Amanda McQuaid, the author of numerous books on herbs, and someone I found not only to be highly intelligent, but also kind and empathetic. I reviewed my herbal treatment protocol with her over the phone. She asked me how I was able to establish such a protocol on my own. I told her simply, "I had to, I was dying."

The symptom I was most anxious to get rid of was the 'malar' rash. Lupus means 'wolf' in Latin. The doctor who named the disease thought his patients looked like they had the bite marks of a wolf. He got that right. I tried everything I could think of within the parameters of my strong belief that medicine should not be harmful in any way. "Do no harm," is the Hippocratic Oath that all doctors take, but most modern medicine falls far short of living up to that.

One of my favorite mixtures was oatmeal and honey. It covered the rash and seemed to calm it down quite a bit. Another was an herb called goldenseal. Goldenseal is brownish green when you add moisture to it. I used to make a paste and apply this to my face. I usually had something on my face, so my family got quite used to seeing me all covered with goop. Many times, I would forget I even had anything on. One day, the doorbell rang. I opened the door to see my five-year-old nephew. He took one look at me and his mouth dropped open. He then took a step back. "What's wrong, DJ?" I asked.

He stammered, "What's on your face...throw-up?"

I laughed, "Just oatmeal." He took a wide circle around me to enter the house. A short while later DJ came to visit again. This time I had goldenseal smeared on the rash and again he acted horrified.

I thought, "What's up? We've been through this before."

This time he squealed, "What's that on your face...poop?"

After ten long years of living with the worst lupus facial rash I had ever seen, one day I read something that would not only take the rash away, it would help me identify the cause of my disease and many other autoimmune diseases.

What I read was this: "The Chinese have made a connection between the face and the stomach." That fascinated me; I had never tried working on my stomach to heal my facial rash. I did some research and tried something I had never tried before. Ten days later, the rash was gone. It has never returned. It wasn't a pill, or an herb, or supplement of any kind. It was a food. Nutrients in that food gave me my first real clue as to what causes this disease. More years would pass before I got my second clue.

Chapter 2 THE DISCOVERY

DNase I

My second clue came one night while I was watching the television show 'Medical Mysteries.' The show was about a young man with some strange and painful symptoms. I usually read while I watch TV, but I closed my book when I heard one of his symptoms. His hands and feet felt at times like someone had poured hot oil over them and placed them in the oven. Once, while visiting with some neighbors outside my home, I felt my own hands start to tingle and then proceed to get progressively warmer, until they felt like they were on fire. It was one of the most painful things I have ever experienced. I went inside and plunged my hands in ice water, where I kept them for the next hour.

It turned out this man had Fabry disease. The similarities with lupus, fibromyalgia, and other autoimmune disorders didn't end there. Some of the other symptoms include: gastrointestinal difficulties, kidney problems, fever, Raynaud's disease-like symptoms with neuropathy, fatigue, nausea, skin rashes, muscle weakness, nervous system problems, periods of intense pain radiating throughout the body, and psychological issues such as depression. Sound familiar to anyone?

It made sense to me that if many of the symptoms of Fabry are the same as other autoimmune diseases, then maybe the cause of Fabry disease would be a clue as to why I was sick. Fabry disease is a genetic disease caused by a lack of the enzyme needed to metabolize lipids (fats). The enzyme is called alpha-galactosidase. It is a mutation in the gene that codes for this enzyme that causes people with Fabry disease to inefficiently break down specific lipids. This leads to an accumulation of these lipids in the blood vessels, kidneys, and the autonomic nervous system. Eventually, this results in impairment of the function of these tissues. I was intrigued. Could lupus and other autoimmune disorders possibly be caused by missing enzymes and the resulting inability to properly break down fats or proteins?

The first clue I had been given was a food that contained enormous amounts of enzymes. The second clue, Fabry disease, also pointed to enzymes. I decided to do additional research. I searched for links to enzymes and lupus and found a study done in Germany that would convince me I was on the right track. When the enzyme deoxcyribonuclease I (DNase I) is removed in mice, they develop lupus! The following article is about the study.

Enzyme Shortage May Lead to Lupus - DNase I
Seppa, N. 2000. *ScienceNews*.

To measure whether ample DNase I can clear the decks and prevent such an onslaught, the researchers created mice that lack the enzyme and compared them with healthy mice. "This is the first genetically defined DNase I-deficient animal," says study coauthor Tarik Moroy, a molecular biologist at the Institute for Cell Biology at the University of Essen.

Moroy and his colleagues examined 69 mice missing the gene that encodes DNase I, as well as 78 others that had a partial enzyme deficiency and 37 that had a full complement of the enzyme. They observed the animals from birth. At eight months, 43 of the 69 totally enzyme-deficient mice showed cell-destroying antibodies in their blood, as did 44 of the 78 partly deficient mice, the researchers report in the June 2000 issue of Nature Genetics. Only nine of the 37 normal mice had any such antibody present.

Indeed, Moroy and his colleagues found that 16 of the 69 fully DNase I-deficient mice and 13 of the 78 partially-deficient mice had kidney inflammation. Only two of the 37 normal mice did.

Journal Reference:
Walport, M.J. 2000. Lupus, DNase and defective disposal of cellular debris. *Nature Genetics* 25:135-136.

After reading this article, I decided I should learn more about this particular enzyme. I discovered that the most well-known job of the enzyme DNase I is to clear out cellular debris and DNA garbage from the body. Without DNase I functioning adequately, the body's own immune cells see leftover cellular debris as a foreign antigen and begin to attack it, forming antibodies against it. These antibodies bind to the debris, which results in the formation of unwanted immune complexes. These immune complexes circulate throughout the bloodstream and lodge themselves in the kidneys, joints, and synovial tissue, causing inflammation and destruction of healthy cells and tissues.

After studying this information, I was so encouraged that I continued researching until I found a corroborating study. This study described two humans with a mutation in the gene that coded for the DNase I enzyme. The mutation in this gene resulted in decreased DNase I enzymatic activity, which the scientists concluded had contributed towards the progression of lupus in the two individuals.

Mutation of DNASE1 in People with Systemic Lupus Erythematosus
Yasutomo, K., T. Horiuchi, S. Kagami, H. Tsukamoto, C. Hashimura, M. Urushihara, Y. Kuroda. 2001. *Nat. Genet.* 28(4):313-4.

Systemic lupus erythematosus (SLE) is a highly prevalent human autoimmune diseases that causes progressive glomerulonephritis, arthritis and an erythematoid rash. Mice deficient in deoxyribonuclease I (DNase1) develop an SLE-like syndrome. Here we describe two patients with a heterozygous nonsense mutation in exon 2 of DNASE1, decreased DNASE1 activity and an extremely high immunoglobulin G titer against nucleosomal antigens. These data are consistent with the hypothesis that a direct connection exists between low activity of DNASE1 and progression of human SLE.

I then found a third study that also implicated the enzyme DNase I as a component in the development of pathogenesis in lupus patients. During an infection, white blood cells form NETs (Neutrophil Extracellular Traps) that ensnare and destroy pathogens. These NETs are made up of DNA and proteins, the exact material that the body is forming antibodies against. Following the infection, DNase I is supposed to decompose these NETs. However, in patients with lupus, DNase I is either absent or defective, so these NETs cannot be degraded properly. This improper degradation of the NETs causes them to become lodged in healthy tissues and results in inflammation and damage. This study identified inefficient removal of extracellular protein NETs as a contributing factor to kidney inflammation (lupus nephritis) in people with lupus, and demonstrated that this was a direct result of impaired DNase I function. Following is an article excerpt from *ScienceDaily* on the study.

Rescue NET for Lupus Patients

ScienceDaily, May 3, 2010

Scientists of the Max Planck Institute for Infection Biology suspected that an immune mechanism that was only recently discovered by them, plays a key role in lupus: During an infection, white blood cells are stimulated and extrude NETs in which they trap and kill pathogens. This NET (an acronym for Neutrophil Extracellular Traps) is composed of exactly those components against which a lupus patient produces antibodies: DNA, as well as proteins of the nucleus and the white blood cells. In co-operation with clinical scientists from the University of Erlangen, the Max Planck scientists could show for the first time that, in contrast to healthy persons, a part of the lupus patients could not degrade NETs after the infection.

The scientists also discovered that NETs are degraded by the enzyme DNase-I, a protein which normally is found in the blood. Lupus patients, however, either lack this enzyme or their DNase-I is blocked. Further examination of this patient group revealed that the remains of NETs together with the auto-antibodies are deposited in the kidneys of systemic lupus erythematosus (SLE) patients. Indeed, the scientists showed a strong correlation between the inability to degrade NETs in lupus and a high risk of kidney failure. These results provide a starting point for the development of a test that might allow an early diagnosis and treatment of these high-risk patients.

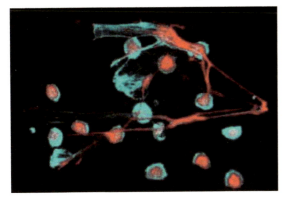

Figure 1: Antibodies (red) on white blood cells are visualized binding to the DNA in NETs (blue) via fluorescent microscopy. (Photo from 2010 *ScienceDaily* article)

Journal Reference:

Hakkim et al. 2010. Impairment of NET degradation is associated with Lupus nephritis. *PNAS* 107(21)9813-9818.

DNase I is found mostly in the pancreas where it is produced. The Department of Biochemistry states, "DNase I as a digestive enzyme that is physiologically regulated is poorly understood. DNase I is mainly responsible for the digestion of dietary DNA before it can be absorbed into the body."

We read above that, *DNase I is responsible for the digestion of dietary DNA before it enters the body*. So, it has another function besides breaking down the NETs and cleaning up cellular debris. The NETs were comprised of the very things that DNase I should have broken down before they entered the bloodstream. If DNase I is missing from the blood, then logically, it would be missing from the pancreas where it originates. This missing enzyme leaves undigested DNA and proteins that should have been broken down during digestion, but were not. Why is the immune system targeting these NETs? Was it only because they were not broken down, or was it because they should not have been there in the first place?

The digestive enzymes in the pancreas include:

- **Lipases**-digest fats, oils and fat-soluble vitamins

- **Amylases**-break down starch molecules into smaller sugars and carbohydrates

- **Proteases**-break down protein into smaller amino acids

- **Ribonucleases**-digest nucleic acids

- **Deoxcyribonuclease I**-digestion of DNA/nuclease

In an additional study from the Department of Biochemistry at Norway's University of Tromsø, it was stated, "Reduction in renal (kidney) DNase I expression and activity is limited to mice and SLE patients with signs of membrane proliferative nephritis, and may be a *critical event* in the development of severe forms of lupus nephritis," (Zykova, 2010).

We know the lack of the single enzyme, DNase I, plays a central role in the development of lupus. If the body lacks DNase I and protease to break down DNA and proteins, would the only ramifications be the development of lupus NETs and the resulting immune response that causes many of the symptoms of lupus? If your body can no longer break down proteins, what other symptoms or diseases could arise?

Chapter 2 THE DISCOVERY

Pancreatic Enzymes, Vitamin B12, and Proteins

How Important are Proteins?

I discovered that proteins, both dietary protein (consumed in the form of eggs, fish, beef, etc.) and body proteins (factors in the blood and tissues), require enzymes to be broken down properly by the body. The first three articles I read had addressed the affect that inefficient enzyme activity had on the body's accumulation of protein in individuals with lupus. Here's where the dietary protein comes in.

Every animal, including humans, must have an adequate source of protein in order to grow and maintain itself. Proteins *yield amino acids,* which are the fundamental structural elements of every cell in the body. There are two major types of amino acids: essential and non-essential. Non-essential amino acids are produced by our bodies, while the essential amino acids must be supplied by our food. The essential amino acids include phenylalanine, valine, threonine, tryptophan, isoleucine, methionine, leucine, and lysine. There is no question that the 'protein' well deserves its name, which is of Greek derivation, meaning "of first importance."

So, pretty important.

Also bound within the dietary proteins we consume in the form of meat, fish, eggs, and dairy, etc., is a vitamin of equal importance, vitamin B12 (also called cobalamin). Animal protein is the only dietary source of B12.

How important is B12? B12 is one of the most biologically active substances known. It is involved in the metabolism of *every cell* in the human body. In addition to playing a major role in DNA replication and the formation of hemoglobin for red blood cells, vitamin B12 is also important for neural cells. It helps form the fatty substance, called 'myelin,' around your nerve cells for protection.

Vitamin B12 is often called the energy vitamin because it helps fat and protein to metabolize in your body. It also plays a major role in the conversion of carbohydrates to glucose—your body's source of fuel. In addition, B12 enables your body to convert fatty acids into energy. It is also a promoter of normal immune function.

If the enzymes necessary to release B12 from protein are not available, then no matter how much protein-bound B12 we consume, we will continue to have a deficiency of B12. The following study concludes *that absorption of vitamin B12 is dependent on the presence of appropriate pancreatic enzymes.*

When the abstract speaks of 'R' proteins, it is referring to the amino acids of which proteins are comprised.

Cobalamin Malabsorption Due to Nondegradation of R Proteins in the Human Intestine

Marcoullis G., Y. Parmentier, J.P. Nicolas, M. Jimenez, P. Gerard. 1980. *J Clin Invest.* 66(3):430–440.

In vivo studies demonstrate that the pancreatic enzymes and the ionic environment in the upper gastrointestinal tract are essential determining factors for transport and absorption of cobalamin in man.

Jejunal fluid was aspirated from healthy human volunteers after administration of cyano [57Co] cobalamin preparations. Immunochemical analysis of the aspirates demonstrated that all isotopic vitamin was transferred to a protein that is identical to the gastric intrinsic factor in terms of molecular mass (57,500), ionic nature (mean pI, 5.09), and reactivity with anti-intrinsic factor sera. However, in the aspirates from patients with exocrine pancreatic dysfunction the vitamin was found to be coupled > 60% to a protein identical to R proteins in terms of molecular mass (125,000), ionic nature (mean pI, 3.51), and reactivity with anti-R protein and anti-intrinsic factor sera. The preferential transfer of cobalamin to R proteins in the patients and to intrinsic factor in healthy subjects was associated, respectively, with low and normal levels of pancreatic enzymes in the intestine and these in turn were paralleled respectively by impaired and normal ileal absorption of cobalamin.

These findings confirm the suggestion that the formation of unabsorbable cobalamin complexes may be the reason of impaired vitamin absorption in exocrine pancreatic insufficiency. Observations made with other selected patients demonstrate: (a) that decreased enzyme activity and nondegradation of R proteins may also be due to nonactivation of pancreatic zymogens in an acidic pH of the intestinal juice the vitamin transported to the jejunum couples to intrinsic factor when pancreatic function is normal, and to intrinsic factor and R protein in exocrine pancreatic insufficiency. The observations made with these selected patients may explain why not all patients with exocrine pancreatic insufficiency develop impaired cobalamin absorption, and also why the malabsorption is corrected by the administration of bicarbonate in certain patients.

The inability to break down dietary proteins into amino acids plays a part in every autoimmune disease, including fibromyalgia, chronic fatigue syndrome (CFS), and lupus. Although CFS and fibromyalgia are not traditionally thought of as autoimmune diseases, we will clearly demonstrate that all these diseases share a common source. Along with lupus sufferers, they are also unable to break down proteins into amino acids. The following study shows that fibromyalgia patients have significantly reduced levels of amino acids.

Altered Amino Acid Homeostasis in Subjects Affected by Fibromyalgia

Bazzichi, L., L. Palego, G. Giannaccini, A. Rossi, F. De Feo, C. Giacomelli, L. Betti, L. Giusti, G. Mascia, S. Bombardieri, A. Lucacchini. 2009. *Clin Bioche*, 42(10-11):1064-70.

The objectives were to evaluate plasma amino acid (AA) concentrations in patients affected by fibromyalgia (FM) and to study the relationships between their levels and FM clinical parameters.

Significant lower plasma taurine, alanine, tyrosine (Tyr), valine, methionine, phenylalanine and threonine concentrations, and the sum of essential AAs were observed in FM patients vs. healthy controls ($P<0.05$). Tyr CAA' ratio and the sum of AAs competing with tryptophan for brain uptake were significantly reduced in FM ($P<0.05$). A significant correlation was found between FM clinical parameters and certain AAs.

Results suggest probable defects of gut malabsorption of certain AAs in FM patients. Moreover, given the reduced Tyr CAA' ratio in FM patients, a possible impairment of the cathecolaminergic system in the FM syndrome may be suggested.

Fibromyalgia patients were found deficient in seven amino acids. For the purposes of our discussion, we will focus on three. They are tyrosine, methionine, and phenylalanine.

Many lupus and fibromyalgia sufferers are also given a diagnosis of chronic fatigue syndrome. Researchers have discovered that chronic fatigue syndrome patients also lack amino acids.

In an open trial published in the Journal of Applied Nutrition, it was found that chronic fatigue syndrome (CFS) patients were deficient in amino acids (Lord, 1994). The highest deficiencies were found in tryptophan and phenylalanine. A full 80% of CFS patients were found to be deficient in tryptophan and 72% had low levels of phenylalanine. The other amino acids found lacking at high levels were taurine, isoleucine, leucine, arginine, and methionine. Just like phenylalanine and tryptophan, these remaining amino acids are found mainly in high protein foods. Leucine, for example, is found mostly in eggs, fish, poultry, dairy, and legumes. Specific foods very high in leucine include chicken, beef, shrimp, black beans, yogurt, and cottage cheese. The following chart is from the trial.

Percentage frequency of amino acids below reference range in 25 CFS subjects (Lord, 1994).

Amino Acid	Percentage	Amino Acid	Percentage
L-Histidine	0	L-Valine	4
L-Threonine	4	L-Lysine	8
L-Methionine	20	L-Arginine	24
L-Leucine	52	L-Isoleucine	60
Taurine	64	L-Phenylalanine	72
L-Tryptophan	80		

Tryptophan is an essential amino acid that is used to make serotonin, a mood-determining brain chemical. Both serotonin and tryptophan shortages have been linked to depression, confusion, insomnia, and anxiety. In the study entitled "Plasma tryptophan and other amino acids in primary fibromyalgia: a controlled study" published in the *Journal of Rheumatology*, researchers found that fibromyalgia patients were also deficient in tryptophan (Yunus, 1992). They state in the conclusion, "Our results suggest that a decreased brain serotonin level, as possibly reflected by decreased transport ratio of plasma tryptophan, may play a pathophysiologic role in primary fibromyalgia."

Fatigue is a part of every autoimmune disease. One important factor of a good night's rest is adequate production of the hormone melatonin. The pineal gland is the primary location for melatonin production. Melatonin is made from tryptophan. The lack of these essential amino acids would account for the depression, insomnia, and anxiety that frequently occur in many autoimmune diseases.

The following study also found that patients with chronic fatigue syndrome (CFS) had significant decreases in phenylalanine and the branched-chain amino acids (Niblett, 2007). There are three branched-chain amino acids; leucine, isoleucine, and valine. The researchers stated that, "Branched-chain amino acids have anabolic and anti-proteolytic effects on muscle protein metabolism and their depletion has been associated with an augmentation in muscle protein proteolysis and a decline in muscle protein levels." This would explain the loss of muscle mass and "wasting" that occurs in CFS.

This paper also states that CFS patients had "a significant decrease in red cell distribution width," and a "significant decrease in succinic acid." Vitamin B12 plays a major role in the formation of red blood cells. B12 is also responsible for the conversion of odd-chain fatty acids into succinate.

A significant decrease in asparagine was also found. Asparagine is a non-essential amino acid. In relation to this, the researchers stated, "The reduction in the urinary output of asparagine in CFS patients noted in this study may be consistent with *impaired protein synthesis*, since asparagine is an important amino acid in protein structures, required for forming glycopeptides."

These are not isolated findings. The researchers stated that, "The majority of studies, including the present investigation, have noted reductions in urine and plasma amino acid levels in patients with CFS compared with healthy controls."

Hematologic and Urinary Excretion Anomalies in Patients with Chronic Fatigue Syndrome

Niblett, S.H., K.E. King, R.H. Dunstan, P. Clifton-Bligh, L.A. Hoskin, T.K. Roberts, G.R. Fulcher, N.R. McGregor, J.C. Dunsmore, H.L. Butt, I. Klienbeg, T.B. Rothkirch. 2007. Exp Biol Med 232(8):1041-9.

Abstract: Patients with chronic fatigue syndrome (CFS) have a broad and variable spectrum of signs and symptoms with variable onsets. This report outlines the results of a single-blind, cross-sectional research project that extensively investigated a large cohort of 100 CFS patients and 82 nonfatigued control subjects with the aim of performing a case-control evaluation of alterations in standard blood parameters and urinary amino and organic acid excretion profiles. Blood biochemistry and full blood counts were unremarkable and fell within normal laboratory ranges. However, the case-control comparison of the blood cell data revealed that CFS patients had a significant decrease in red cell distribution width and increases in mean platelet volume, neutrophil counts, and the neutrophil-lymphocyte ratio. Evaluation of the urine excretion parameters also revealed a number of anomalies. The overnight urine output and rate of amino acid excretion were both reduced in the CFS group ($P < 0.01$). Significant decreases in the urinary excretion of asparagine ($P < 0.0001$), phenylalanine ($P < 0.003$), the branch chain amino acids ($P < 0.005$), and succinic acid ($P < 0.0001$), as well as increases in 3-methylhistidine ($P < 0.05$) and tyrosine ($P < 0.05$) were observed. It was concluded that the urinary excretion and blood parameters data supported the hypothesis that alterations in physiologic homeostasis exist in CFS patients.

Conclusions: The results of this study revealed that patients with CFS/ME had anomalies in blood parameters, urine excretion volume, and urinary excretion of amino acids compared with age- and sex-matched nonfatigued controls. Reductions in overnight urinary output and a generalized depletion in the rate of amino acid excretion, in particular, depletions in the excretion of branched chain amino acids, were the most prominent alterations observed. These findings indicated significant disturbance to amino acid and nitrogen metabolism and homeostasis. Further investigation into the mechanisms underlying these changes and their etiologic and clinical significance is warranted.

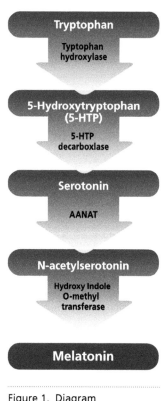

Figure 1. Diagram demonstrating the production of serotonin and melatonin from the amino acid tryptophan

To the left is a chart showing the relationship between the amino acid tryptophan and subsequent production of serotonin and melatonin.

Lying at the very center of your body's ability to create energy is your mitochondria. Mitochondria are structures that are found inside virtually every cell in your body. They are the 'power houses' of the cell. One of the most essential substances for the mitochondria is carnitine. Carnitine is a critical compound your body produces using dietary amino acids. It is used by the mitochondria of cells to produce energy and in the export of toxic waste materials from the cell. Your body manufactures carnitine from the essential amino acids lysine and methionine. As cited in the previous studies, methionine was one of the essential amino acids that fibromyalgia and CFS patients lacked. Again, these amino acids are derived from dietary proteins. They are the same proteins your body can't break down if you have an autoimmune disease. Low levels of the carnitine compound, acylcarnitine, in the blood or muscles of people with CFS/FMS, have been found in the following studies:

1. Plioplys, A.V., S. Plioplys. 1997. Amantadine and L-Carnitine Treatment of Chronic Fatigue Syndrome. Neuropsychobiology 35(1):16-23.

2. Kuratsune, H., K. Yamaguti, M. Takahashi, et al. 1994. Acylcarnitine Deficiency in Chronic Fatigue Syndrome. Clinical Infectious Disease 18(3 Supplement 1): S62-S67.

3. Reuter, S.E., A.M. Evans. 2010. Long-chain Acylcarnitine Deficiency in Patients with Chronic Fatigue Syndrome. Potential Involvement of Altered Carnitine Palmitoyltransferase-I Activity. Journal of Internal Medicine:1365-2796.

As with carnitine, the essential amino acid methionine is also needed to produce glutathione. You may have heard of this "rock star" of antioxidants. It is an integral part of the body's detoxification system. It helps the mitochondria avoid or repair damage that would normally lead to mitochondrial dysfunction and cell death. Methionine is a precursor for cysteine, and cysteine is a precursor for glutathione.

The lack of methionine would lead to a deficiency in glutathione. In the study entitled "Serum antioxidants and nitric oxide levels in fibromyalgia: a controlled study" glutathione levels were found to be "significantly lower in fibromyalgia patients than in controls," (Sendur, 2009). Low glutathione levels are a common finding in people suffering from autoimmune diseases. In the study "Correlation of lipid peroxidation and glutathione levels with severity of systemic lupus erythematosus: a pilot study from single center" the researchers concluded that, "A significant correlation between plasma GSH (glutathione) and SLE severity exists that may aid evaluation of the disease severity and usefulness of the treatment of SLE," (Tewthanom, 2008).

In addition to carnitine and glutathione, another critical component necessary for the proper functioning of the mitochondria is Coenzyme Q10 (CoQ10). It acts as an essential cofactor to produce adenosine triphosphate (ATP), which is the currency of energy in the body. To produce ATP, mitochondria need certain essential raw nutrients, such as carnitine and CoQ10. CoQ10 also functions as an antioxidant.

A recent study found that plasma CoQ10 was significantly lower in chronic fatigue syndrome patients than in normal control patients (Maes, 2009). It stated, "Up to 44.8% of patients with ME/CFS had values beneath the lowest plasma CoQ10 value detected in the normal controls…"

CoQ10 is a fat-soluble compound synthesized by the body and also consumed in the diet. A report from Iowa State University lists beef, chicken, pork, and fish as the foods with the highest levels of CoQ10. In a healthy person, CoQ10 can be synthesized, but it requires the presence of one of two amino acids we have found lacking in CFS and fibromyalgia, phenylalanine or tyrosine.

According to the Linus Pauling Institute's Micronutrient Information Center at Oregon State University, one of the major steps involved in biosynthesis of coenzyme Q10 uses either tyrosine or phenylalanine for synthesis of the benzoquinone structure (Higdon, 2003).

Tyrosine is derived from phenylalanine, and phenylalanine is found in high protein foods. Without the ability to break down high protein foods, you would not have the necessary amino acids to produce CoQ10.

A word of caution: The lack of amino acids found in CFS and fibromyalgia are a result of the inability to digest dietary proteins. If you are unable to digest proteins, you would also be unable to properly metabolize the amino acids of which proteins are comprised. The previous study "Cobalamin Malabsorption Due to Nondegration of R Proteins in the Human Intestine" showed that pancreatic enzymes are necessary to degrade R proteins (amino acids). The inability to digest proteins and amino acids is what led to the unbroken down bits of protein and DNA in the bloodstreams of lupus patients. The immune system targets these proteins and forms immune complexes, which then become lodged in healthy organs and tissues. Taking additional amino acids in supplement form would lead to an increased risk of disease. This is evident in the findings from a study entitled "Intermediary Metabolism of Phenylalanine and Tyrosine in Diffuse Collagen Diseases" (Nishimura, 1959). When lupus patients were given supplements of tyrosine and phenylalanine, the supplements "unfailingly aggravated both clinical signs and laboratory data of collagen disease."

It is important to note that the previous studies found low levels of numerous amino acids in the plasma of fibromyalgia and chronic fatigue syndrome patients. If fibromyalgia and chronic fatigue syndrome patients are not breaking down proteins into amino acids, then they are also unable to release B12. In the next section, we will identify symptoms and findings of fibromyalgia, chronic fatigue syndrome, and other autoimmune diseases that are a result of protein and B12 deficiency.

The Importance of B12 and Protein

The fibromyalgia message boards are abuzz about a video of a leading researcher on fibromyalgia, Dr. Patrick Wood. Dr. Wood is a respected authority on the causes and treatment of fibromyalgia. He is head of the Louisiana State University (LSU) Fibromyalgia Research Department and Clinic, and is a current scientific advisor for the National Fibromyalgia Association. His innovative research has caused him to be twice recognized by the American National Institutes for Health.

Dr. Wood has made some amazing discoveries associated with brain abnormalities in people suffering with fibromyalgia. It has cost millions of dollars, but the results have shed some light on the disease process involved. The brains of people with fibromyalgia have reduced levels of dopamine. Additionally, he has found that fibromyalgia patients have changes in their spinal cords and low-levels of iron. The members of the fibromyalgia boards are ecstatic. This is the first time that there has been actual evidence of a fundamental difference between the brain of a fibromyalgia patient and that of a healthy individual.

I watched the video with interest. What is the connection between the lack of sufficient enzymes, inability to break down proteins, and reduced levels of dopamine? Since I found his research credible, I knew there had to be one. I must admit that as my husband watched the video, he got a little wide eyed. Did this new research somehow negate what I knew to be true or would it add credence to it? Within the hour, I knew the answer.

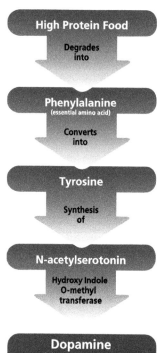

The brain cells, which manufacture dopamine, depend on the essential amino acid phenylalanine. Phenylalanine is found in high protein foods. People with fibromyalgia, chronic fatigue syndrome, lupus, and other autoimmune diseases are unable to break down high protein foods because they lack the enzymes to do so. Therefore, they cannot release essential amino acids. In the previous studies, it was shown that fibromyalgia and chronic fatigue patients were deficient in phenylalanine.

Figure 2. Diagram illustrating the relationship between dopamine synthesis and dietary proteins

What about low iron levels and the spinal cord changes?

Fibromyalgia patients would not have sufficient iron if they were lacking protein and B12. B12 and iron are often mentioned together, although one is a vitamin and the other is a mineral. The dietary sources of B12 and iron are often the same, so that deficiencies in the two may occur at the same time. Vitamin B12 is derived in the diet only from animal sources and is very abundant in meat. Meat also contains high amounts of iron. Other animal sources that are abundant in both B12 and iron include poultry, pork, and seafood. If you lack the enzymes to break down these proteins, then it would make sense that B12, along with iron, would not be available to the body.

In addition, the same enzymes that break down dietary proteins (proteases) are also responsible for regulating iron absorption in the body. Without these enzymes, the body would not be able to properly metabolize iron. The following abstract concludes that the serine protease TMPRSS6 is an essential component of a pathway that detects iron deficiency and regulates iron absorption in the body.

New Insights Into Intestinal Iron Absorption
Hörl, W.H. 2008. Nephrol. Dial. Transplant. 23(10):3063-3064.

…Du et al. described the novel and exciting finding that the transmembrane serine protease 6 (TMPRSS6) senses iron deficiency [1]. In their study, Du et al. described a mutant mouse, which is characterized by progressive loss of body hair and microcytic anaemia. The phenotype was found to result from reduced intestinal iron absorption caused by high levels of hepcidin. Iron deprivation and anaemia suppressed hepcidin mRNA levels in the livers of wild-type mice, whereas high mRNA levels persisted in the livers of anaemic mutant mice. The high hepcidin levels in the mutant mice resulted from a splice defect in the Tmprss6 gene. This suggests that TMPRSS6 physiologically downregulates hepcidin mRNA transcription and thus promotes iron uptake [1].

Take home message: Iron deficiency activates the serine protease TMPRSS6. The protease then inhibits hepcidin transcription and thereby allows intestinal iron absorption and cellular iron release.

Low iron is a common finding in autoimmune disease. Symptoms of iron deficiency include anemia, fatigue, rapid heartbeat, inability to concentrate, disturbed sleep, severe menstrual pain and bleeding, cracks in the corners of the mouth, mouth ulcers, and hair loss (as was shown in the study).

Low iron would also lead to another common condition found in fibromyalgia and other autoimmune diseases; restless legs syndrome. A study published in the Journal of Clinical Sleep Medicine found that 33% of people with fibromyalgia also had restless legs syndrome. This is not surprising since restless legs syndrome has been linked in studies to both low iron and dopamine. Following is an abstract of one such study.

Dopamine and Iron in The Pathophysiology of Restless Legs Syndrome (Rls)
Allen, R. 2004. Sleep Med. 5(4):385-91.

Background and Purpose: The evaluation of the pathophysiology of restless legs syndrome (RLS) stems largely from recognition of the information provided by both pharmacological treatment of the disorder and the secondary forms of the disorder. This article examines the pathophysiological implications of each of these clinical aspects of RLS.

Patients and Methods: The article reviews the existing literature in relation to possible pathology suggested by the clinical data. It will then explore other data supporting each of the possible pathologies and examine the relationships between these pathologies.

Results: The pharmacological treatment data strongly support a dopaminergic abnormality for RLS. Other pharmacological data and some imaging data also support this, although the data are not entirely consistent. The secondary forms of RLS strongly support an iron deficiency abnormality for RLS, further documented by several other studies. Some animal studies have shown a relation between iron deficiency and dopaminergic abnormalities that have some similarity to those seen in the RLS patient.

Conclusions: It is concluded that there may be an iron-dopamine connection central to the pathophysiology of RLS for at least some if not most patients with this disorder.

Dr. Wood also identified changes in the spinal cord. According to the National Institutes of Health, subacute combined degeneration of the spinal cord is caused by a vitamin B12 deficiency.

Subacute Combined Degeneration
National Institutes of Health, 25 June 2009

Subacute combined degeneration of the spinal cord is a disorder that involves weakness, abnormal sensations, mental problems, and vision difficulties.

Causes: Subacute combined degeneration of the spinal cord is caused by a vitamin B12 deficiency.

Subacute combined degeneration primarily affects the spinal cord, but it can also damage the brain, the nerves of the eye, and the peripheral (body) nerves. At first, the disease damages the covering of the nerves (the myelin sheath). It later affects the entire nerve cell.

How a lack of vitamin B12 damages nerves is unclear. However, experts believe the lack of this vitamin causes abnormal fatty acids to form around cells and nerves.

You have a higher risk for this condition if you cannot absorb vitamin B12 from the intestines or if you have:

- Pernicious anemia
- Disorders of the small intestine, including Crohn's disease
- Malabsorptive conditions, which can occur after gastrointestinal surgery

Symptoms: These symptoms slowly get worse and are usually felt on both sides of the body. Abnormal sensations (tingling and numbness), weakness of the legs, arms, middle of the body, or other areas

Other symptoms include:

- Clumsiness, stiff, or awkward movements
- Unsteady gait and loss of balance
- Change in mental state such as memory problems, irritability, apathy, confusion, or dementia
- Decreased vision
- Depression
- Sleepiness
- Speech impairment (possible)

Even if your serum (blood) levels of B12 are normal, you may still have a B12 deficiency. Your cellular levels are often lower than your serum levels. *More than 60% of chronic fatigue and fibromyalgia patients show low levels of B12 in cerebrospinal fluid, where these degenerative changes in the spinal cord are taking place.*

I often hear, "I've had my B12 levels checked. They are normal." Let's take a closer look at the meaning of the word 'normal.' A study done at Tufts University may indicate that B12 deficiency is far more widespread than previously believed (McBride, 2000). The study looked at 3,000 individuals and found that 40% of the participants had low B12 values. Additionally, the study used 258 pg/mL as their criterion for a 'low level.' Other countries, however, use a much higher B12 level (approximately 500-600 pg/mL) to determine a deficiency. Of critical note; 500-600 pg/mL is the level at which memory loss, lethargy, and dementia can occur.

The levels of serum vitamin B12 considered 'normal' in the United States are vastly lower than that of other countries like Japan and some European countries. American medical opinion defines blood levels lower than 200 pg/mL as an indication of deficiency. This number is based on the level associated with the most severe manifestation of deficiency, which is pernicious anemia (abnormally formed red blood cells). Physicians in Japan and other countries consider blood levels of 500-1300 pg/mL to be the normal range. If you are within the "normal" range in the U.S., you have a severe deficiency-enough to cause pernicious anemia. Instead of just 60%, what would the B12 deficiency rate have been in the cerebrospinal fluid of fibromyalgia and chronic fatigue syndrome patients had they used the higher standards of these other countries?

One surprising fact mentioned in the Tufts University study was that the participants were eating foods rich in vitamin B12, but their bodies were not absorbing the vitamin. As was concluded in the Cobalamin Malabsorption study, the absorption of B12 is dependant on the presence of appropriate pancreatic enzymes. This is very important to keep in mind as we move forward. No amount of vitamin B12 will reverse the symptoms of autoimmune disease, unless the mechanism your body has to absorb it is restored. The problem lies in the metabolism of B12, not just in the amount consumed. Absorption also depends on whether it is in natural or supplement form.

According to the Lupus Foundation of America, in about half of those with lupus, the disease attacks the brain and spinal cord. Science has not yet been able to provide an explanation for this. The following abstract shows that spinal cord changes can occur even with so-called normal levels of B12 in the blood.

Subacute Combined Degeneration with High Serum Vitamin B12 Level and Abnormal Vitamin B12 Binding Protein. New Cause of an Old Syndrome

Reynolds E.H., T. Bottiglieri, M. Laundy, J. Stern, J. Payan, J. Linnell, J. Faludy 1993.
Arch Neurol. Jul;50(7):739-42.

Subacute combined degeneration of the spinal cord due to vitamin B12 deficiency invariably has been associated with a low serum vitamin B12 level. We describe a young man who presented with a unique syndrome of subacute combined degeneration associated with high serum vitamin B12 level, low red blood cell vitamin B12 level, and an abnormal plasma vitamin B12-binding protein. Uptake of cobalamin by his leukocytes in vitro was inhibited by his own but not by normal control plasma. Intensive hydroxocobalamin (vitamin B12) treatment was associated with clinical and electrophysiologic recovery accompanied by normalization of mean corpuscular volume, red blood cell vitamin B12 level, plasma homocysteine, and urinary methylmalonic acid. The subacute combined degeneration was probably precipitated by treatment with folic acid as the significance of his high serum vitamin B12 level was not apparent when he first presented with megaloblastic anemia 3 years earlier. To our knowledge, this is the first example of neurologic disease associated with high serum vitamin B12 level and provides further evidence that sometimes a serum vitamin B12 level may not be a reliable guide to vitamin B12 deficiency.

All of Dr. Wood's findings: reduced levels of dopamine, low iron, and spinal cord changes, can be clearly and completely explained by the body's lack of pancreatic enzymes (proteases) that break down dietary proteins. In addition, this would also explain the brain and spinal cord changes that often occur in lupus.

We will now examine the findings of another well-known and respected researcher in fibromyalgia, Dr. Manuel Martinez-Lavin, M.D. I will let his research speak for itself.

A Novel Holistic Explanation for the Fibromyalgia Enigma: Autonomic Nervous System Dysfunction

Martinez-Lavín, M. 2001. *Fibromyalgia Frontiers* 10(1).

This article discusses scientific evidence supporting the notion that all fibromyalgia (FM) features can be explained on the basis of autonomic (sympathetic) nervous system dysfunction. On this basis, a holistic approach for FM treatment is proposed.

My first argument is that FM is a multi-system illness. This means that FM symptoms are not limited to the muscles as the name fibromyalgia may suggest. It is obvious that this illness also produces dramatic manifestations in different organs and systems of the body. The most frequent associated complaints are: fatigue, sleep disorders, morning stiffness, headache, a numbness and tingling feeling in the extremities, restless legs, anxiety, dryness in the mouth, cold-clammy hands, irritable bowel, mental fogginess, and cystitis. So, any valid theory attempting to explain FM mechanisms should first give a coherent explanation for the presence of these disparate symptoms in the same patients. When we started our FM research at the National Cardiology Institute of Mexico, our working hypothesis was that all of the above-mentioned features could be explained on the basis of autonomic nervous system dysfunction.

What Is the Autonomic Nervous System?

The autonomic nervous system (ANS) is the portion of the nervous system that controls the function of the different organs and systems of the body. For instance, it regulates body temperature, blood pressure, heartbeat rate, and bowel and bladder tone, among many other variables. It is "autonomic" because our mind does not govern its performance; rather, it works below the level of consciousness. One striking characteristic of this system is the rapidity and intensity of the onset of its action and its dissipation. Centers located in the central nervous system (brain stem, hypothalamus, and thalamus) and in the spinal cord activate the ANS. These centers also receive input from the limbic system and other higher brain areas. This means that the ANS is the interface between mind and body functions. These connections enable the ANS to be the main component of the stress response system in charge of fight-or-flight reactions.

The ANS works closely with the endocrine system (the hormonal system), particularly the hypothalamic-pituitary-adrenal axis. Another endocrine axis closely related to the ANS involves growth hormone secretion.

The peripheral autonomic system is divided into two branches; sympathetic and parasympathetic. These two branches have antagonistic effects on most bodily functions, and their proper balance preserves equilibrium. Thus, the ANS represents the ying-yang concept of ancient eastern cultures. Sympathetic activation prepares the whole body for fight or flight in response to stress or emergencies; in contrast, parasympathetic tone favors digestive functions and sleep. The sympathetic autonomic branch extends from the brain stem to the spinal cord and features rich sympathetic nerve tissue in the neck and pelvic areas (important facts for FM research). From the spinal cord, the sympathetic nervous system goes to our internal organs and to the extremities. At the skin level, sympathetic activity induces cold clammy hands, mottled skin, and piloerection (goose flesh).

The action of the two branches of the ANS is mediated by neurotransmitters. Adrenaline (also known as norepinephrine) is the predominant sympathetic neurotransmitter whereas acetylcholine acts in the parasympathetic periphery.

Until recently, the action of this extremely dynamic ANS has been difficult to assess in clinical practice. Changes in breathing pattern, mental stress, or even posture alter immediately and completely the sympathetic/parasympathetic balance. Nevertheless, with the introduction of a new powerful cybernetic technique named heart rate variability analysis, the outlook has changed dramatically.

What is Heart Rate Variability Analysis?
This technique is based on the fact that the heart rate is not uniform but varies continuously from beat to beat by a few milliseconds. The periodic components of this endless heart rate variation are dictated by the antagonistic impulses that the sympathetic and parasympathetic branches have on the heart. Cybernetic recording of this constant variability is able to estimate both sympathetic and parasympathetic activity. The elegance of this method resides in the fact that all measurements are derived from electrocardiograms, so patients are subjected to no discomfort whatsoever.

Heart rate variability analysis is not a test that a patient can readily obtain from practicing physicians. So far, this test is largely confined to research centers.

Our Research on Fibromyalgia
We have used heart rate variability analysis to estimate ANS function in patients with FM. We have found that such patients have changes consistent with relentless hyperactivity of their sympathetic nervous system which continues 24 hours a day. Very interestingly, in a different study, we subjected FM patients to a simple stress test which involved having them stand up. Their overworked sympathetic nervous system became unable to further respond meaning that the system was already exhausted.

It is known that as we stand up, blood tends to pool in the lower parts of the body. In normal circumstances, there is an immediate sympathetic surge that compensates for this blood shift and maintains normal blood circulation to the head. People with FM clearly have an abnormal response, and their sympathetic nervous system fails to respond properly. It is pertinent to mention that researchers from different parts of the world have confirmed these abnormal heart rate variability findings in patients with FM.

Based on this research, we proposed that dysautonomia (the medical term for ANS dysfunction) is frequent in patients with FM. Such dysautonomia can be characterized as a sympathetic nervous system that is persistently hyperactive but hypo-reactive to stress. Furthermore, we propose that such dysautonomia explains all FM features. Our ANS findings fully agree with previous ground-breaking research on sleep disorders and hormonal abnormalities in FM.

Dysautonomia Explains All FM Features

Sympathetic hypo-reactivity provides a coherent explanation for the constant fatigue and other symptoms associated with low blood pressure, such as dizziness, fogginess, and faintness. This phenomenon can be compared to what would happen to a constantly forced engine that becomes unable to speed up in response to further stimulation.

Relentless sympathetic hyperactivity also explains the sleep disturbances associated with FM. It is known that parasympathetic tone predominates during deep sleep stages and that seconds before awakening episodes there is a sympathetic surge. Our concurrent studies of polysomnography and heart rate variability analyses have shown that FM people have relentless nocturnal sympathetic hyperactivity associated with constant arousal and awakening episodes.

Sympathetic hyperactivity may also explain the cold, clammy hands (pseudo Raynaud's phenomenon) and the constant dryness in the mouth often seen in persons with FM. Investigators who have directly studied irritable bowel syndrome and interstitial cystitis have also reported alterations which are consistent with sympathetic hyperactivity.

About the Author: Manuel Martínez-Lavín, M.D. graduated as a physician from the National University of Mexico. He did his postgraduate training in Internal Medicine at St. Louis University in Missouri and in Rheumatology at Scripps Clinic in La Jolla, California. He is certified in Internal Medicine and Rheumatology by the American Board of Internal Medicine. He is currently Chief of the Rheumatology Department at the National Cardiology Institute of Mexico. He has published over 60 research articles in scientific, peer-reviewed journals. His research interest focuses on cardiovascular involvement in rheumatic diseases.

Dr. Lavin concluded, "Dysautonomia explains all FM features."

What is dysautonomia? Dysautonomia is a dysfunction of the autonomic nervous system. The Merck Manual states, "The autonomic nervous system is the part of the nervous system that supplies the internal organs, including the blood vessels, stomach, intestine, liver, kidneys, bladder, genitals, lungs, pupils, and muscles of the eye, heart, and sweat, salivary, and digestive glands. The autonomic nervous system controls blood pressure, heart and breathing rates, body temperature, digestion, metabolism (thus affecting body weight), the balance of water and electrolytes (such as sodium and calcium), the production of body fluids (saliva, sweat, and tears), urination, defecation, sexual response, and other processes.

A dysfunction in the autonomic nervous system (dysautonomia) can cause dizziness or light-headedness due to excessive decrease in blood pressure when a person stands (orthostatic hypotension). People may sweat less or not at all and thus become intolerant of heat. The eyes and mouth may become dry. After eating, a person with dysautonomia may feel prematurely full or even vomit because the stomach empties very slowly (gastroparesis). Some people pass urine involuntarily (urinary incontinence), often because the bladder is overactive. Other people have difficulty emptying the bladder (urine retention) because the bladder is underactive. Constipation may occur, or control of bowel movements may be lost. The pupils may not dilate and narrow (constrict) as light changes."

Just as with Dr. Wood's findings, Dr. Lavin's research can be clearly explained by the body's inability to break down dietary protein and release B12.

"The prototype of dysautonomia is the ancient scourge of beriberi, a nutritional deficiency disease due to excess of simple carbohydrate and concomitant vitamin B1 deficiency. In the early stages this results in loss of functional efficiency in the central control mechanisms of the autonomic nervous system. If the nutritional deficiency continues, there is gradual degeneration of the system," (Wikipedia, 2011b).

No other B vitamin is more dependent on its fellow B vitamins than B1. If you are deficient in B12, you will not be able to absorb B1. It will be *excreted in the urine.*

Following are two abstracts showing the relationship between a deficiency of vitamin B12 and a dysfunction of the autonomic nervous system (dysautonomia).

Rare Sensory and Autonomic Disturbances Associated with Vitamin B12 Deficiency

Puntambekar, P., M.M. Basha, I.T. Zak, R. Madhavan. 2009. *J Neurol Sci* 15:287(1-2):285-7.

Vitamin B12 deficiency is an important nutritional disorder causing neurological manifestations of myelopathy, neuropathy and dementia. Sub-acute combined degeneration (SCD) with involvement of the posterior columns in the cervical and thoracic cord is a common presentation of this disorder. In this case report, we describe a 43 year old woman with pernicious anemia and myelopathy with atypical clinical features. The patient presented with motor symptoms, a sensory level and bladder dysfunction. She had severe autonomic disturbances including an episode of unexplained bronchospasm, which has not been previously reported as a manifestation of vitamin B12 deficiency. We review the literature regarding these rarely reported features of vitamin B12 deficiency, and discuss aspects of management of this reversible condition. We emphasize the importance of awareness of autonomic disturbances in B12 deficient individuals

Autonomic Dysfunction and Hemodynamics in Vitamin B12 Deficiency

Beitzke, M, P. Pfister, J. Fortin, F. Skrabal. 2002. *Auton Neurosci.* 18:97(1):45-54.

Orthostatic hypotension in patients with cobalamin (Cbl) deficiency has been reported previously in isolated cases but we are not aware of detailed systematic studies of hemodynamic and autonomic nervous system function in patients with cobalamin deficiency. We investigated hemodynamic and autonomic responses to 60 degrees passive head up tilt (HUT) in 21 patients with vitamin B12 deficiency, 21 healthy age-matched control subjects and 9 age-matched patients with diabetes mellitus (DM) and established diabetic neuropathy. To systematically assess hemodynamic and autonomic nervous system function, we performed measurements of heart rate, beat-to-beat systolic and diastolic blood pressure, stroke index, cardiac index, total peripheral resistance index, total power, low (LF) and high (HF) frequency oscillatory component of heart rate variability, LF/HF ratio and spontaneous baroreflex sensitivity. As compared to controls, we found a significant fall of systolic blood pressure during 60 consecutive beats directly after head up tilt; furthermore, a significantly blunted fall of stroke index, cardiac index and a lack of increase of total peripheral resistance index for the duration of tilt in patients with diabetes mellitus and in patients with vitamin B12 deficiency. As compared to controls, we observed an altered response of spectral indices of sympathetic activation and vagal withdrawal and an impaired modulation of baroreflex sensitivity during head up tilt suggestive of a complex modification in the neural control activities in patients with cobalamin deficiency, which was comparable to that observed in patients with diabetes mellitus and established autonomic neuropathy. The results suggest that vitamin B12 deficiency causes autonomic dysfunction with similar hemodynamic consequences and patterns of autonomic failure as seen in diabetic autonomic neuropathy. Defective sympathetic activation may be the cause for orthostatic hypotension, which is occasionally seen in patients with vitamin B12 deficiency. It is concluded that patients with orthostatic hypotension should be screened for cobalamin deficiency.

As we have discussed, B12 is vital in many bodily processes, including the synthesis of myelin (which surrounds nerve cells). B12 is also essential to the development of red blood cells and DNA. Dietary protein is the only natural food source of B12 for humans. Since digestive enzymes are required to release B12 from the protein before it can be absorbed into the body, a problem with one of these enzymes could potentially result in a serious B12 deficiency. As mentioned previously, severe depletion of B12 manifests as pernicious anemia. This occurs at the level that the U.S. defines as a deficiency (200 pg/mL). Long before anemia becomes apparent, however, other conditions manifest themselves. Symptoms such as muscle fatigue, shaking, burning sensations, pins and needles, irrational anger, memory loss, impaired mental function, and Alzheimer's may become evident. These neurological symptoms manifest themselves at approximately 500-600 pg/mL.

According to WebMD, the same symptoms of motor nerve and sensory nerve damage attributed to dysautonomia can also be caused by a vitamin B12 deficiency. These symptoms include: weakness, muscle atrophy, twitching, paralysis, pain sensitivity, numbness, tingling, pinching, burning, and abnormal or hyperactive reflexes.

The Mayo Clinic states, "Studies have shown that a deficiency of vitamin B12 can lead to abnormal neurologic and psychiatric symptoms. These symptoms may include ataxia (shaky movements and unsteady gait), muscle weakness, spasticity, incontinence, hypotension (low blood pressure), vision problems, dementia, psychoses, and mood disturbances."

This is a list of known symptoms of Vitamin B12 deficiency:

- Numbness and tingling
- Anemia
- Ataxia (irregularity of muscular action)
- Concentration difficulties
- Pale lips
- Dementia
- Depression
- Personality changes
- Apathy
- Psychosis
- Aversion to meat
- Canker sores
- Seizures
- Nervousness
- Weakness/loss of muscle strength
- Inadequate melatonin metabolism leading to disruptive sleep patterns
- Impaired memory and memory loss
- Dizziness
- Abnormal or hyperactive reflexes
- Abnormal coordination
- Impaired perception of deep touch, pressure and vibration
- Rapid heartbeat
- Loss of appetite
- Sudden electric-like shocks going down the spine
- Confusion
- Fever
- Irritability
- Lightheadedness
- Tiredness
- Pallor
- Dyspnea
- Hair loss
- Burning tongue
- Nerve pain
- Brittle nails
- Jaundice
- Enlargement of the mucous membranes of the mouth tongue, and stomach
- Frequent upper respiratory infections
- Diarrhea
- Nausea
- Gastrointestinal symptoms
- Decrease or abolishment of deep muscle-tendon reflexes

As Dr. Lavin demonstrated, dysautonomia certainly does explain many of the features of fibromyalgia. Indeed, these same symptoms occur in many other autoimmune diseases, such as multiple sclerosis and myasthenia gravis. The lack of B12 has been shown to have a direct link to dysautonomia. Dr. Lavin also stated, "The action of the two branches of the ANS is mediated by neurotransmitters. Adrenaline is the predominant sympathetic neurotransmitter, whereas acetylcholine acts in the parasympathetic periphery."

To produce adrenaline and acetylcholine to regulate the ANS (autonomic nervous system), it would be necessary for you to be able to properly break down proteins. *Vitamin B12 and folate are required for the synthesis of choline before becoming acetylcholine.*

In the previous studies shown on fibromyalgia and chronic fatigue syndrome and amino acids, it was concluded that both fibromyalgia and chronic fatigue sufferers showed significantly lower levels of amino acids. One of the amino acids found to be deficient was phenylalanine. Adrenaline is derived from the essential amino acid phenylalanine. If you are unable to produce dopamine, you would also be unable to produce adrenaline, as was shown in the dopamine diagram.

Autonomic Dysfunction and Chronic Fatigue Syndrome

The following study abstract found that chronic fatigue syndrome patients also have dysautonomia or a dysfunction of the autonomic nervous system. The researchers stated, "Our data show a clear and significant association between CFS (identified using the established Fukuda criteria) and the symptoms of autonomic dysfunction (identified using the COMPASS score.)"

Symptoms of Autonomic Dysfunction in Chronic Fatigue Syndrome

Newton, J.L., O. Okonkwo, K. Sutcliffe, A. Seth, J. Shin, D.E.J. Jones. 2007.QJM 100(8):519-526.

Background: Chronic fatigue syndrome (CFS) is common and its cause is unknown.

Aim: To study the prevalence of autonomic dysfunction in CFS, and to develop diagnostic criteria.

Design: Cross-sectional study with independent derivation and validation phases.

Methods: Symptoms of autonomic dysfunction were assessed using the Composite Autonomic Symptom Scale (COMPASS). Fatigue was assessed using the Fatigue Impact Scale (FIS). Subjects were studied in two groups: phase 1 (derivation phase), 40 CFS patients and 40 age- and sex-matched controls; phase 2 (validation phase), 30 CFS patients, 37 normal controls and 60 patients with primary biliary cirrhosis.

Results: Symptoms of autonomic dysfunction were strongly and reproducibly associated with the presence of CFS or primary biliary cirrhosis (PBC), and correlated with severity of fatigue. Total COMPASS score >32.5 was identified in phase 1 as a diagnostic criterion for autonomic dysfunction in CFS patients, and was shown in phase 2 to have a positive predictive value of 0.96 (95%CI 0.86–0.99) and a negative predictive value of 0.84 (0.70–0.93) for the diagnosis of CFS.

Discussion: Autonomic dysfunction is strongly associated with fatigue in some, but not all, CFS and PBC patients. We postulate the existence of a 'cross-cutting' aetiological process of dysautonomia-associated fatigue (DAF). COMPASS >32.5 is a valid diagnostic criterion for autonomic dysfunction in CFS and PBC, and can be used to identify patients for targeted intervention studies.

Autonomic dysfunction is also found in rheumatoid arthritis and lupus. The following study concludes, "SLE (lupus) and RA are associated with severe autonomic dysfunction."

Cardiac Autonomic Dysfunction in Patients with Systemic Lupus, Rheumatoid Arthritis and Sudden Death Risk

Milovanovi, B., L. Stojanovi, N. Milievik, K. Vasi, B. Bjelakovi, M. Krotin . 2010. Srp Arh Celok Lek. 138(1-2):26-32.

Introduction: The manifestations of autonomic nervous system (ANS) dysfunction in autoimmune diseases have been the subject of many studies. However, the published results pertaining to such research are controversial. Sudden cardiac death due to fatal arrhythmias is frequent in patients with systemic lupus erythematosus (SLE) and rheumatoid arthritis (RA).

Conclusion: SLE and RA are associated with severe autonomic dysfunction and the presence of significant risk predictors related to the onset of sudden cardiac death.

Is Sjögren's Syndrome Caused by Dysautonomia?

Government researchers are asking that very question. Sjögren's syndrome is another co-concurring disease with many of the other autoimmune illnesses. The main symptoms of Sjögren's syndrome involve the mucous membranes. Sjögren's syndrome is named after Henrik Sjögren (1899-1986), the Swedish ophthalmologist who first described it, and is marked by extremely dry mouth and dry eyes. In a study to be conducted by the National Institutes of Health, researchers are challenging the current understanding that Sjögren's stems from the autoimmune-driven destruction of the exocrine glands, leading to their hypofunction and symptoms of dryness (National Institutes of Health Clinical Center, 2010). They state, "The existing evidence, however, does not fully support this assumption and cannot explain the underlying pathogenic mechanisms for Sjögren's for the following reasons:

- Discordance between severely affected function and abundance of histologically normal and ex vivo functional salivary glands.
- At least 20% of patients have no evidence of systemic autoimmunity.
- Animal models of Sjögren's develop glandular dysfunction long before they develop autoimmunity.
- Dryness and related symptoms respond poorly to immunosuppressives, but fairly well to secretagogues such as polocarpine."

Secretion of saliva is under the control of the autonomic nervous system, which controls both the volume and type of saliva secreted. It makes sense that a dysfunction of the salivary glands could be associated with a dysfunction in the autonomic nervous system, by which they are controlled.

This following study shows that researchers are finding a link between patients with Sjögren's syndrome and a dysfunction of the autonomic nervous system.

Autonomic Nervous Symptoms in Primary Sjögren's Syndrome: A Follow-up Study

Mandl, T., V. Granberg, J. Apelqvish, P. Wollmer, R. Manthrope, L.T.H. Jacobsson. 2008. Autonomic nervous symptoms in primary Sjögren's syndrome. *Rheumatology* 47:914-919

Objective: Signs of autonomic dysfunction (AD) have been reported in patients with primary SS (pSS) while the presence of associated symptoms has not been systematically studied. Therefore, the aims of this study were (i) to assess the presence and severity of various AD symptoms in pSS patients and (ii) to relate AD symptoms to other clinical features of pSS.

Methods: Thirty-eight pSS patients and 200 population-based controls were studied for presence and severity of AD symptoms using the Autonomic Symptom Profile (ASP), a validated self-completed questionnaire evaluating various AD symptoms. In addition, patients were investigated by three different objective autonomic nervous function tests.

Conclusions: pSS patients showed subjective and objective signs of both a parasympathetic and a sympathetic dysfunction. However, AD symptoms showed limited associations with objective autonomic nervous function as well as other clinical features of the disease.

In an additional study done at Malmö University Hospital's Department of Rheumatology in Sweden, researchers concluded, "Both objective and subjective symptoms of parasympathetic and sympathetic dysfunction were seen in primary Sjögren's syndrome patients. Autonomic dysfunction symptoms were significantly associated with fatigue, anxiety, and depression," (Mandl, 2009). If there is a connection between Sjögren's and the autonomic nervous system, then we should be able to find that Sjögren's is linked to a B12 deficiency. Following is a study which discusses the link.

Sjögren's Syndrome Associated with Vitamin B12 Deficiency

Wegelius, O., F. Fyhrquist, P.L. Adner. 1987. *Scan Jnl Rheumt.* 16(1):184-190.

Three patients showing Sjögren's syndrome in association with macrocytic anemia due to vitamin B12 deficiency are described. Antibodies to parietal cells, intrinsic factor and salivary protein were investigated; positive test results were obtained in different combinations. Addisonian pernicious anemia as well as vitamin B12-malabsorption because of anti-intrinsic factor antibodies in gastric juice and/or malabsorption due to changes in the intestinal wall induced by Sjögren's syndrome are possible etiological factors. A case of Sjögren's syndrome associated with positive anti-parietal cell antibodies and histaminerefractory achylia is also reported. The concurrence of these two diseases known to be associated with autoimmune responses suggests the possibility of similar pathogenesis.

A vitamin B12 deficiency can also lead to the sore mouth and tongue often associated with Sjögren's. It is periodically accompanied by a bitter or metallic taste (Cigna, 2010). B12 deficiency impairs DNA synthesis, which affects all proliferating cells. Without B12, developing cells in the bone marrow cannot divide normally to form mature red blood cells. Instead, they become unusually large and misshapen, and most never leave the bone marrow. This results in a specific type of anemia, a deficiency of red blood cells. A similar accumulation of large abnormal cells lining the digestive tract can cause a sore mouth and tongue.

The abstract below found that 25% of the Sjögren's patients tested had low B12. If they were tested at the current level of B12 deficiency for the U.S. though, the number may not reflect the actual deficiency rate. Just as in fibromyalgia, the study found that Sjögren's patients lack iron. *Fifty-one percent of 1 degree Sjögren's patients were deficient in iron.*

If Sjögren's is caused by dysautonomia, then we would also expect Sjögren's patients to have a higher risk of developing thyroid problems. This would be true, since both of the thyroid hormones (thyroxine and triiodothyronine), are also derived from tyrosine, just as adrenaline is. Adrenaline is one of the neurotransmitters that regulates the autonomic nervous system. In addition to low B12 and low iron, the following abstract found that 33% of the patients tested had thyroid disease and 30% had autoimmune thyroiditis or Hashimoto's.

Iron and Vitamin Deficiencies, Endocrine and Immune Status in Patients with Primary Sjögren's Syndrome

Lundström, I.M., F.D. Lindström. 2001. Oral Dis. 7(3):144-9.

Objectives: To study the prevalence of iron and vitamin deficiencies, endocrine disorders and immunological parameters in patients with primary Sjögren's syndrome (1 degree SS).

Design And Subjects: At the time of the establishment of the diagnosis of 1 degree SS in 43 consecutive patients, a clinical examination including haematological analyses was performed. The patients' medical records were also reviewed.

Setting: Patients referred for diagnosis to The University Hospital, Linköping, a secondary or tertiary referral hospital serving the middle part of southern Sweden.

Results: In total, current or previously treated iron and vitamin deficiencies were registered for 63% of the 1 degree SS patients (iron 51%, vitamin B12 25%, folate 9%). Current low ferritin was noted in 24%, low iron saturation in 37%, decreased vitamin B12 in 13% and folate in 9%. Thyroid disease was found in a total of 33% and 30% had had autoimmune thyroiditis. Three patients (7%) had verified diabetes mellitus. Erythrocyte sedimentation rate (ESR) was raised in 65% of the patients and 84% had a polyclonal increase of Ig. Rheumatoid factor (RF) was detected in 85%, antinuclear antibody (ANA) in 74%, anti-SS-A in 88% and anti-SS-B in 73% of the patients.

Conclusion: Iron and vitamin deficiencies and thyroid diseases are common in patients with 1 degree SS. Since these disorders often are treatable and may affect the patients' distress as well as their immune and exocrine function, an active, recurrent search for deficiencies, endocrine diseases and other frequently recorded disorders is recommended.

The study also detected rheumatoid factor in 85% of the Sjögren's patients. What is rheumatoid factor? Rheumatoid factor is currently defined as an autoantibody directed against an organism's own tissues. These antibodies join to form immune complexes. These are the same immune complexes we saw in the previous study entitled "Rescue Net for Lupus Patients". We discovered that the immune system was targeting unbroken down protein fragments and DNA. We will learn more about what else the immune system is actually targeting in autoimmune disease as we move forward.

The following study identifies pancreatic insufficiency in not only Sjögren's syndrome, but in rheumatoid arthritis as well.

Pancreatic Duct Antibodies and Subclinical Insufficiency of the Exocrine Pancreas in Sjögren's Syndrome

D'Ambrosi, A., A. Verzola, P. Buldrini, C. Vavalle, S. Panareo, S. Gatto, R. La Corte, L. Vicentini, A. Boccafogli, R. Scolozzi. 1998. Recenti Prog Med 89(10):504-9.

Abstract: In previous studies we reported evidence of subclinical exocrine pancreatic insufficiency in primary or secondary Sjögren's syndrome (SSI, SSII) and rheumatoid arthritis (RA). In present study we evaluated the occurrence of pancreatic duct antibodies (PDA), and their relationship to exocrine pancreatic function in 36 women. Of these patients, 12 were classified as SSI, 12 as SSII, and 12 as RA. Exocrine pancreatic function was evaluated using the Secretin-Caerulein test (S.Cae test). The indirect immunofluorescent technique was used to evaluate patient sera for PDA. S.Cae test results, compared to controls, showed a statistically significant decrease in duodenal juice volumes, bicarbonates and enzymes in 58.3% of SSI, in 58.3% of SSI and in 30% of RA, according to our previous trials. PDA were found in two patients, the former with SSI and the latter with SSII, both asymptomatic with regard to pancreatic diseases but with impaired exocrine pancreatic function as evaluated by S.Cae test. We discuss the possible causes of these results.

Thyroid Deficiency, Amino Acids, and B12

People with vitamin B12 deficiency, anemia, or low thyroid function all complain about the same thing. All three conditions cause fatigue. In pernicious anemia, red blood cells are abnormally formed due to an inability to absorb B12. According to a study titled: *Anemia in Hypothyroidism*, "Pernicious anemia occurs *20 times more frequently* in patients with hypothyroidism than generally," (Antonijević, 1999).

In order to make the thyroid hormones thyroxine and triiodothyronine, you would need to be able to digest dietary proteins. Both of these thyroid hormones are tyrosine-based. Tyrosine is an amino acid that is derived from the break down of dietary proteins. As we have discussed, it is also needed to make dopamine and adrenaline.

Figure 3. Diagram demonstrating tyrosine production from the essential amino acid phenylalanine

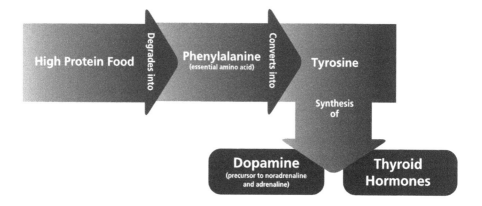

As the diagram above demonstrates, both of the adrenal hormones, adrenaline and noradrenaline, are also derived from the essential amino acid phenylalanine. This would explain why autoimmune sufferers may be given corticosteroid or other anti-inflammatory medications to help alleviate some of their symptoms. Lack of these adrenal hormones could also account for some of the fatigue found in autoimmune disease.

Following are two studies showing that vitamin B12 deficiency is common in hypothyroidism. The first study shows an approximately 40% prevalence of B12 deficiency in hypothyroid patients. The second study concludes that 28% of patients had low levels. While the deficiencies found in these studies are remarkable, these numbers likely would have been much higher if a more appropriate set of criteria had been used. First, they tested serum (blood) levels. Cellular levels are often much lower. Second, they used an extremely low level to determine a deficiency—133 pg/mL. Remember, at more than three times that level (500 pg/mL), you will start to see disease symptoms such as memory loss, lethargy, and dementia. In the U.S., current levels used to determine a deficiency are set at 200 pg/mL, the level at which severe changes in the blood cells occur.

Vitamin B12 Deficiency Common in Primary Hypothyroidism

Jabbar, A., A. Yawar, S. Waseem, N. Islam, N. Ul Haque, L. Zuberi, A. Khan, J. Akhter. 2009. J Pak Med Assoc 59(2):126.

Objective: To assess the prevalence and clinical features of B12 deficiency in hypothyroid patients and to evaluate clinical response in symptoms to B12 replacement therapy.

Methods: One hundred and sixteen hypothyroid patients from our endocrine clinic were evaluated for signs and symptoms of vitamin B12 deficiency. Laboratory parameters including Haemoglobin (Hb), MCV, Vitamin B12 levels and presence of anti thyroid antibodies were analyzed. Patients with low B12 levels were treated with parenteral intramuscular vitamin B12 monthly, and monitored for improvement of symptoms.

Results: A total of 116 patients (95 females and 21 males) were evaluated. Forty six (39.6%) hypothyroid patients had low vitamin B12 levels. Males and females had the same prevalence of B12 deficiency. Generalized weakness, impaired memory, depression, numbness and decreased reflexes were more frequently noted in B12 deficient patients, but failed to achieve statistical significance when compared with B12 sufficient patients. The mean Hb in B12 deficient group was 11.9 +/- 1.6 mg/dl and 12.4 +/- 1.7 mg/dl in the B12 sufficient group, however the mean MCV did not differ in the two groups. Patients with B12 deficiency did not have a higher prevalence of anaemia. Thyroid antibodies were checked in half the patients and 67% had positive titers for anti thyroid antibodies. Prevalence of vitamin B12 deficiency did not differ in patients with positive antibodies (43.2%) compared to those with negative antibodies (38.9%) (p= 0.759). Twenty four hypothyroid patients with B12 deficiency received intramuscular vitamin B12 injections monthly and improvement in symptoms was noted in 58.3% of these subjects. Additionally, 21 subjects complained of symptoms consistent with B12 deficiency but who had normal range B12, levels and were prescribed monthly B12 injections and 8 (40%) had good subjective clinical response at 6 months.

Conclusions: There is a high (approx 40%) prevalence of B12 deficiency in hypothyroid patients. Traditional symptoms are not a good guide to determining presence of B12 deficiency. Screening for vitamin B12 levels should be undertaken in all hypothyroid patients, irrespective of their thyroid antibody status. Replacement of B12 leads to improvement in symptoms, although a placebo effect cannot be excluded, as a number of patients without B12 deficiency also appeared to respond to B12, administration.

Prevalence and Evaluation of B12 Deficiency in Patients with Autoimmune Thyroid Disease

Ness-Abramof, R., D.A. Nabriski, L.E. Braveman, L. Shilo, E. Weiss, T. Rashef, M.S. Shapiro, L. Shenkman. 2006. Am J Med Sci 332(3):113-22.

Background: Patients with autoimmune thyroid disease (AITD) have a higher prevalence of pernicious anemia compared with the general population. Clinical signs of B12 deficiency may be subtle and missed, particularly in patients with known autoimmune disease. We assessed the prevalence of vitamin B12 deficiency in patients with AITD and whether their evaluation may be simplified by measuring fasting gastrin levels.

Methods: Serum B12 levels was measured in 115 patients with AITD (7 men and 108 women), with a mean age of 47 +/- 15 years. In patients with low serum B12 levels (< or =133 pmol/L), fasting serum gastrin and parietal cell antibodies (PCA) were measured.

Results: Thirty-two patients (28%) with AITD had low B12 levels. Fasting serum gastrin was measured in 26 and was higher than normal in 8 patients. PCA were also measured in 27 patients with B12 deficiency and were positive in 8 patients. Five patients with high gastrin levels underwent gastroscopy with biopsy, and atrophic gastritis was diagnosed in all. The prevalence of pernicious anemia as assessed by high serum gastrin levels in patients with low B12 was 31%.

Conclusions: Patients with AITD have a high prevalence of B12 deficiency and particularly of pernicious anemia. The evaluation of B12 deficiency can be simplified by measuring fasting serum gastrin and, if elevated, referring the patient for gastroscopy.

Vitamin B12, Proteins, and Multiple Sclerosis

I recently read an article written by Julie Stachowiak, Ph.D. (Stachowiak, 2008). I thought she conveyed the connection to multiple sclerosis (MS) and B12 deficiency so well, that I am including parts of her article so that you can read it in her own words.

"When I dabbled in vegetarianism (I was even a pretty strict vegan for about a year), I was able to tell you that vegetarians need to supplement with B12. I couldn't really tell you why. I also didn't ever take a supplement. Now that I have multiple sclerosis, I am pretty shocked to learn that a vitamin B12 deficiency is higher in people with MS than those that don't have MS."

She continued, "Studies have reported a significantly higher rate of vitamin B12 deficiency in people with MS than in people without MS, which is suspected to be due to problems with binding and transport of vitamin B12 (meaning that the body does not process B12 efficiently). One study found low B12 levels in the cerebrospinal fluid of people with MS, although their blood levels were normal. People with vitamin B12 deficiency have destruction of both the myelin and the underlying axon. If the deficiency is severe, there can be serious brain damage, causing MS-like symptoms. Even when people have slight B12 deficiency, they may exhibit symptoms like fatigue, depression, and memory loss. Vitamin B12 helps maintain the myelin sheath by playing a crucial role in the metabolism of fatty acids essential for the maintenance of the myelin."

Well said. Don't you think?

As Dr. Stachowiak stated, vitamin B12 helps maintain the myelin sheath by playing a crucial role in the metabolism of fatty acids essential for the maintenance of the myelin. The study entitled "Deficiencies of polyunsaturated fatty acids and replacement by nonessential fatty acids in plasma lipids in multiple sclerosis" found that, "All omega 3 acids were subnormal" in the MS patients compared to healthy controls (Holman, 1989). Additionally, the researchers determined that, "Loss of polyunsaturated fatty acids and replacement by nonessential acids lowered mean chain length and raised mean melting point significantly, suggesting that lowered membrane fluidity was only partially compensated by endogenous synthesis of lower-melting, nonessential acids."

Recent research has found that so-called 'normal' levels of B12 are significantly associated with a greater severity of white matter lesions. They are called white matter lesions because of their color. The whiteness is caused by the myelin sheath that covers the axons. The conclusion of the following abstract states, "Our results indicate that vitamin B12 status in the normal range is associated with white matter lesions, especially periventricular lesions. Given the absence of an association with cerebral infarcts, we hypothesize that this association is explained by effects on myelin integrity in the brain rather than through vascular mechanisms." (Myelin is the insulating lining of nerve fibers, which aids in quick and accurate transmission of electrical current/messages between nerve cells).

Plasma Vitamin B12 Status and Cerebral White-matter Lesions

de Lau, L.M., A.D. Smith, H. Refsum, C. Johnston, M.M. Breteler. 2009.
J Neurol Neurosurg Psychiatry 80(2) :149-57.

Background and Objectives: Elevated homocysteine has been associated with a higher prevalence of cerebral white-matter lesions and infarcts, and worse cognitive performance. This raises the question whether factors involved in homocysteine metabolism, such as vitamin B(12), are also related to these outcomes. This study examined the association of several markers of vitamin B(12) status with cerebral white-matter lesions, infarcts and cognition.

Methods: The study evaluated the association of plasma concentrations of vitamin B(12), methylmalonic acid, holotranscobalamin and transcobalamin saturation with cerebral white-matter lesions and infarcts at baseline and cognition at baseline and during follow-up among 1019 non-demented elderly participants of the population-based Rotterdam Scan Study. Analyses were adjusted for several potential confounders, including homocysteine and folate concentration.

Results: Poorer vitamin B(12) status was significantly associated with greater severity of white-matter lesions, in particular periventricular white-matter lesions, in a concentration-related manner. Adjustment for common vascular risk factors (including blood pressure, smoking, diabetes and intima media thickness) did not alter the associations. Adjustment for homocysteine and folate modestly weakened the associations. No association was observed for any of the studied markers of vitamin B(12) status with presence of brain infarcts and baseline cognition or cognitive decline during follow-up.

Conclusions: These results indicate that vitamin B(12) status in the normal range is associated with severity of white-matter lesions, especially periventricular lesions. Given the absence of an association with cerebral infarcts, it is hypothesised that this association is explained by effects on myelin integrity in the brain rather than through vascular mechanisms.

It is a common misconception that white matter lesions are what differentiate MS from other autoimmune diseases. In his article "MRI white matter lesions: does it represent MS?" Dr. Nitin Sethi, Assistant Professor of Neurology at New York-Presbyterian Hospital states, "Thus, it is important to remember that a person who is really noted to have white matter lesions on a brain MRI does not necessarily have MS. White matter lesions can be seen in numerous other conditions and they are more commonly seen as we grow older."

If the white matter lesions found in MS are indeed due to a lack of vitamin B12, then we should be able to find the same white matter lesions in all of the diseases we have been discussing, since they also lack vitamin B12. In addition to MS, white matter lesions can also be found in lupus, chronic fatigue syndrome, Sjögren's syndrome, rheumatoid arthritis, myasthenia gravis, celiac disease, and other diseases as well. The following study demonstrates their presence in Sjögren's syndrome.

Cerebral White Matter Lesions in Primary Sjögren's Syndrome: A Controlled Study

Coates, T., J.P. Slavotinek, M. Rischmueller, D. Schultz, C. Anderson, M. Dellamelva, M.R. Sage, T.P. Gordon. 1999. J. Rheumatol. 26(6):1301-5.

Objective: To determine the prevalence of neurological and magnetic resonance imaging (MRI) abnormalities in a well defined population of unselected patients with primary Sjögren's syndrome (SS) and age and sex matched healthy patients.

Methods: Thirty patients with SS and 29 age and sex matched controls were examined by a neurologist and subsequently underwent MRI scanning with a 1.0 Tesla Siemens Impact MR scanner. Scans were graded by a neuroradiologist blinded to the clinical status of each subject. The number and location of white matter lesions > 3 mm in long axis (to exclude non-specific perivascular changes) were recorded for each subject.

Results: There was a significant increase in lesions detected by MRI in SS patients versus controls ($p = 0.02$) including deep white matter lesions ($p = 0.03$) and subcortical white matter lesions ($p = 0.02$). The presence of white matter lesions did not correlate with serum IgG or rheumatoid factor levels, or with presence of anticardiolipin antibodies. No subjects had symptoms or signs of serious neurological disease including multiple sclerosis, and corpus callosal lesions commonly seen in multiple sclerosis were notably absent in this study.

Conclusion: Cerebral white matter lesions detected by MRI are more frequent in patients with primary SS than control subjects, yet do not appear to be associated with significant clinical manifestations. Although the pathological nature of these lesions is yet to be defined, their presence should not be over-interpreted.

Following are three studies that clearly implicate B12 deficiency in multiple sclerosis:

Multiple Sclerosis Associated with Vitamin B12 Deficiency

Reynolds, E.H., J.C. Linnell, J.E. Faludy. 1991. Arch Neurol. 48(8):808-11.

Abstract: We describe 10 patients with a previously unreported, to our knowledge, association of multiple sclerosis and unusual vitamin B12 deficiency. The clinical features and the age at presentation were typical of multiple sclerosis, with eight cases occurring before age 40 years, which is a rare age for vitamin B12 deficiency. Nine patients had hematologic abnormalities, but only two were anemic. All six patients examined had low erythrocyte cobalamin levels. Only two patients had pernicious anemia; in the remaining patients the vitamin B12 deficiency was unexplained. A vitamin B12 binding and/or transport is suspected. The nature of the association of multiple sclerosis and vitamin B12 deficiency is unclear but is likely to be more than coincidental. Further studies of vitamin B12 metabolism, binding, and transport in multiple sclerosis are indicated, as these cases may offer a clue to the understanding of a still mysterious neurologic disorder.

Vitamin B12 Metabolism in Multiple Sclerosis

Reynolds, E.H., T Bottiglieri, M. Laundy, R.F. Crellin, S.G. Kirker. 1992. Arch Neurol. 49(6):649-52.

We have previously described 10 patients with multiple sclerosis (MS) and unusual vitamin B12 deficiency. We have therefore studied vitamin B12 metabolism in 29 consecutive cases of MS, 17 neurological controls, and 31 normal subjects. Patients with MS had significantly lower serum vitamin B12 levels and significantly higher unsaturated R-binder capacities than neurological and normal controls, and they were significantly macrocytic compared with normal controls. Nine patients with MS had serum vitamin B12 levels less than 147 pmol/L and, in the absence of anemia, this subgroup was significantly macrocytic and had significantly lower red blood cell folate levels than neurological and normal controls. Nine patients with MS had raised plasma unsaturated R-binder capacities, including three patients with very high values. There is a significant association between MS and disturbed vitamin B12 metabolism. Vitamin B12 deficiency should always be looked for in patients with MS. The cause of the vitamin B12 disorder and the nature of the overlap with MS deserve further investigation. Coexisting vitamin B12 deficiency might aggravate MS or impair recovery from MS.

Vitamin B12 and its Relationship to Age of Onset of Multiple Sclerosis

Sandyk, R., G.I. Awerbuch. 1993. *Int J Neurosci.* 71(1-4):93-9.

Attention has been focused recently on the association between vitamin B12 metabolism and the pathogenesis of multiple sclerosis (MS). Several recent reports have documented vitamin B12 deficiency in patients with MS. The etiology of this deficiency in MS is unknown. The majority of these patients do not have pernicious anemia and serum levels of the vitamin are unrelated to the course or chronicity of the disease. Moreover, vitamin B12 does not reverse the associated macrocytic anemia nor are the neurological deficits of MS improved following supplementation with vitamin B12. It has been suggested that vitamin B12 deficiency may render the patient more vulnerable to the putative viral and/or immunologic mechanisms widely suspected in MS. In the present communication, we report that serum vitamin B12 levels in MS patients are related to the age of onset of the disease. Specifically, we found in 45 MS patients that vitamin B12 levels were significantly lower in those who experienced the onset of first neurological symptoms prior to age 18 years (N = 10) compared to patients in whom the disease first manifested after age 18 (N = 35). In contrast, serum folate levels were unrelated to age of onset of the disease.

As vitamin B12 levels were statistically unrelated to chronicity of illness, these findings suggest a specific association between the timing of onset of first neurological symptoms of MS and vitamin B12 metabolism. In addition, since vitamin B12 is required for the formation of myelin and for immune mechanisms, we propose that its deficiency in MS is of critical pathogenetic significance.

A common symptom of multiple sclerosis is nystagmus. Nystagmus is involuntary, rapid repetitive movements of the eyes. To an onlooker, it might resemble the eye movements of someone looking at the scenery from the window of a moving train. However, it may be unnoticeable to the person with nystagmus. The following abstract shows the connection to nystagmus and lack of vitamin B12.

Downbeat Nystagmus Indicates Cerebellar or Brain-stem Lesions in Vitamin B12 Deficiency

Mayfrank, L., U. Thoden. 1986. *J Neurol* 233(3):145-8.

Abstract: Two cases of vitamin B12 deficiency caused by gastric atrophy are described. Together with the neuropsychiatric features usually associated with this condition, a downbeat nystagmus syndrome was observed. It is concluded that vitamin B12 deficiency may also result in lesions to those cerebellar or brain-stem structures that are generally assumed to cause downbeat nystagmus.

We have identified a lack of amino acids in the pathogenesis of fibromyalgia, chronic fatigue syndrome, Sjögren's, and hypothyroidism. We can also find this same lack of amino acids in multiple sclerosis patients. Following is a quote from an article in US News & World Report (University of Illinois at Chicago, 2011).

"'Multiple sclerosis is associated with reduced levels of an important neurotransmitter, noradrenaline. There is a lot of evidence of damage to the Locus Coeruleus (LC) in Alzheimer's and Parkinson's disease, but this is the first time it has been demonstrated that there is stress involved to the neurons of the LC of MS patients, and that there is a reduction in brain noradrenaline levels,' said the study's first author, Paul Polak, a research specialist at the University of Illinois at Chicago." The study was published online February 4, 2011 in Brain.

In order to produce noradrenaline you would need to be able to digest dietary proteins. This adrenal hormone is derived from tyrosine. Tyrosine is an amino acid that is derived from the essential amino acid phenylalanine. Phenylalanine is found in high protein foods.

The following study shows that phenylalanine, tyrosine, and tryptophan were all "found to be diminished" in the cerebrospinal fluid of patients with MS.

Plasma and Cerebrospinal Fluid Tryptophan in Multiple Sclerosis and Degenerative Diseases

Monaco, F., S. Fumero, A. Mondino, R. Mutani. 1979. J. Neurol. Neurosurg. Psychiatry 42:640-641.

Tryptophan and competing neutral amino acid levels were found to be diminished in the plasma of patients with multiple sclerosis and degenerative diseases, the greatest decrease being of tryptophan. Cerebrospinal fluid tryptophan was decreased in multiple sclerosis and motor neurone disease, while leucine and valine were increased. These changes might lead to decreased synthesis of brain serotonin and brain proteins. The ratio between neutral amino acids and tryptophan might be used as an ancillary test in the screening of degenerative diseases.

Results:Tryptophan, leucine, isoleucine, valine, tyrosine, and phenylalanine were all diminished in the plasma of patients with multiple sclerosis (Table) but by far the greatest decrease was in the tryptophan level (t> 11), as well as tyrosine and phenylalanine (t>4), all of them having a P value of <0.001.

The lack of phenylalanine, as shown in the previous study, would lead to a lack of dopamine (see graph on page 46). Low dopamine levels are associated with the following symptoms (Dellwo, 2011):

- Stiff, rigid, achy muscles
- Cognitive impairment
- Impaired motor skills
- Tremors
- Inability to focus attention
- Poor balance and coordination
- Strange walking pattern (gait), frequently with small steps

Subacute degeneration of the spinal cord and dysautonomia would account for many of the symptoms of multiple sclerosis. We have demonstrated that subacute combined degeneration of the spinal cord is caused by a vitamin B12 deficiency. Studies have shown a significantly higher rate of vitamin B12 deficiency in people with MS. Dysautonomia is caused by a vitamin B12 deficiency and lack of the neurotransmitters adrenaline and acetylcholine, which regulate the autonomic nervous system. Vitamin B12 and folate are required for the synthesis of choline before becoming acetylcholine. Adrenaline is produced by the body when the body modifies noradrenaline. MS patients have been found to lack noradrenaline, as well as B12. This would lead to both subacute combined degeneration of the spinal cord and dysautonomia.

The following study on multiple sclerosis and autonomic dysfunction (dysautonomia) states, "*Ninety percent* of the patients had symptoms related to autonomic dysfunction…"

Autonomic Dysfunction in Multiple Sclerosis: Correlation with Disease-Related Parameters

Gunal, D.I., N. Afsar, T. Tanridag, S. Aktan. 2002. *Eur Neurol.* 48(1):1-5.

Abstract: Cardiovascular autonomic functions were investigated in a prospective, controlled study of 22 consecutive relapsing-remitting multiple sclerosis (MS) patients and 22 healthy subjects using 5 simple noninvasive tests and sympathetic skin response testing. Tests included the heart rate response to deep breathing, valsalva maneuver and standing, blood pressure response to standing and sustained hand grip, and were graded according to the Ewing and Clark classification as early, definite or severe impairment. The relationship between autonomic dysfunction and disease-related parameters such as the expanded disability status scale (EDSS) and disease duration was studied. Ninety percent of the patients had symptoms related with autonomic dysfunction, and 45.5 % had abnormal results in cardiovascular autonomic function testing with 4 patients also having abnormal sympathetic skin responses. Statistical analysis indicated that patients with a long disease duration rather than high EDSS carried a risk of autonomic involvement in MS. Both parasympathetic and sympathetic functions were impaired and this could have been easily overlooked by a standard EDSS follow-up. In this regard, autonomic function testing seems necessary in order to detect subclinical changes in MS patients and should be considered in outcome measures.

An additional study found that, "Clinical and laboratory evidence of AD (autonomic dysfunction) was found in 84% and 56% of MS patients respectively. The researchers concluded, "Furthermore, AD appears more closely related to axonal loss, as demonstrated by spinal cord atrophy, than to demyelinating lesions."

Autonomic Dysfunction in Multiple Sclerosis: Cervical Spinal Cord Atrophy Correlates

de Seze, J., T. Stojkovic, J.Y. Gauvrit, D. Devos, M. Ayachi, F. Cassim, T. Saint Michel, J.P. Pruvo, J.D. Guieu,
P. Vermersch. 2001. *J Neuol.* 248(4):297-303.

Abstract: Autonomic dysfunction has rarely been studied in patients suffering from multiple sclerosis (MS). Some hypotheses have concerned the pathophysiology, especially with regard to a possible spinal cord origin. However, there have been no previous studies on autonomic dysfunction in MS and spinal cord lesions. This study assessed the frequency of autonomic dysfunction (AD) in MS and the correlation to spinal cord magnetic resonance imaging (MRI) findings. We prospectively studied 75 MS patients (25 with relapsing-remitting forms, 25 with secondary progressive forms and 25 with primary progressive forms). We performed sympathetic skin response, R-R interval variability and orthostatic hypotension testing. Spinal cord MRI was performed to detect demyelinating lesions (sagittal and axial plane) or spinal cord atrophy. Clinical and laboratory evidence of AD was found in 84% and 56% of MS patients, respectively. The correlation of the latter with disability was evaluated using the Extended Disability Status Scale. AD was more frequent in primary progressive MS than in the other two forms. AD was correlated with spinal cord cross-sectional area reduction but not with spinal cord hyperintensities. This study confirms that the frequency of AD in MS, especially in primary progressive forms, has until now been underestimated. Furthermore, AD appears to be more closely related to axonal loss, as demonstrated by spinal cord atrophy, than to demyelinating lesions.

Lack of proteases would also lead to another symptom commonly associated with MS and other autoimmune conditions; chronic itching. As the following information shows, proteases play an important part in mediating the itch response. Proteases are also called proteinases. In the study entitled "Proteinase-Activated Receptor-2 Mediates Itch: A Novel Pathway for Pruritus in Human Skin" the conclusion states, "In summary, proteinases appear to play an important role as itch mediators in human skin very likely by activating PAR-2. The existence of a histamine-independent, proteinase-dependent, and PAR-2 mediated pathway provides a new link that may lead to beneficial therapies for pruritus and cutaneous inflammation," (Steinhoff, 2003).

It really doesn't matter what the symptom or the finding is in autoimmune disease, they can all be traced back to missing protease. Even the most obscure, puzzling findings, are now easily explained. One of these puzzling findings in MS has been that MS patients generally don't get gout. Here is a quote from a 1998 study (Hooper, 1998):

"A possible association between multiple sclerosis (MS), the disease on which EAE (experimental allergic encephalomyelitis) is modeled, and uric acid is supported by the finding that patients with MS have significantly lower levels of serum uric acid than controls. In addition, statistical evaluation of more than 20 million patient records for the incidence of MS and gout (hyperuricemic) revealed that the two diseases are almost mutually exclusive, raising the possibility that hyperuricemia may protect against MS."

Gout is caused by an excess of uric acid. Uric acid is the final break down product of DNA. Remember the first lupus study and the picture of the unbroken-down protein particles and DNA in the lupus patients' bloodstream? This was a result of a lack of the enzyme DNase 1, whose job it is to break down DNA and proteins. The lack of DNase 1 would lead to low levels of uric acid. This would explain the study finding that MS and gout are "almost mutually exclusive."

We will discuss additional findings on multiple sclerosis in the sections on homocysteine and tumor necrosis factor.

Arthritis and Adequate Protein Digestion

Lita Lee, Ph.D., a chemist, enzyme nutritionist, and nutritional counselor, explained the connection well when she wrote, "All forms of arthritis involve abnormal calcium metabolism. Ninety-nine percent of the body calcium is (or should be) in the bones and teeth. The other one percent, found in the blood, is just as important because it is essential in the blood clotting mechanism, muscle and nerve function, vitamin D function, and the function of hormones that control calcium metabolism (called parathyroid hormones). Of the one percent of calcium in the blood, half is protein-bound and half is ionized. Both require *adequate protein digestion*. If you are deficient in protein because you can't digest it, you cannot carry protein-bound calcium. If you lack optimum acidity from inadequate digestion of protein, you will not have enough ionized calcium. In either case, you are a candidate for arthritis.

The abnormal deposit of calcium is one of the factors involved in arthritis and arthritic inflammation. Soft tissue, any kind of body tissue other than bones and teeth, is a target for depositing calcium. Wherever this happens, pathology occurs: in the joints, around inflamed areas (osteoarthritis), in the arteries (arteriosclerosis), in the kidneys (kidney stones), in the soft lenses of the eyes (cataracts), in the brain (stroke) and so on," (Lee, 2009).

The inability to carry protein-bound calcium would explain the low levels of vitamin D found throughout autoimmune disease. Without blood borne calcium, you would not be able to properly metabolize vitamin D. The problem lies in the binding and transport, just as with vitamin B12. In autoimmune disease, taking additional vitamin D or calcium in supplement form, that you are not able to properly metabolize, would just give your body more vitamin D and calcium to deposit in your joints and tissues. It may also lead to another autoimmune disease called sarcoidosis. Sarcoidosis is an inflammatory condition that produces tiny lumps of cells called granulomas in various organs of the body. These granulomas clump together into large or small groups, resulting in organ damage. Dysregulated calcium and vitamin D metabolism are well-recognized features of sarcoidosis.

Low levels of vitamin D and calcium can cause muscle weakness and bone pain. Muscle weakness, pain, muscle cramps, and twitching are all associated with vitamin D and calcium deficiency. Vitamin D plays a role in regulating cellular processes in the nervous system and muscle tissue. Without proper levels of vitamin D, electrical impulses along nerve pathways may begin to misfire, causing muscles at different locations in the body to contract and relax. Proper muscle function can be restored, without the risk of additional disease symptoms, by restoring your body's ability to carry protein-bound calcium.

"Osteoporosis is a common feature in adults with Rheumatoid Arthritis," according to the National Rheumatoid Arthritis Society (Litwic, 2010). In a 2006 British study, it was found that people with RA are 50% more likely to develop osteoporosis (van Staa, 2006). The study, of approximately 30,000 people with RA, found that the risk of osteoporosis existed even if no other risk factor, such as the long-term use of corticosteroids or smoking, was present. In fact, the risk posed by RA alone was as great as the risk caused by taking corticosteroids.

When the blood cannot carry protein-bound calcium because it lacks protein, it withdraws the necessary calcium from the bones to maintain homeostasis or internal balance. The bones need sufficient calcium to develop and maintain bone structure.

The inability to metabolize vitamin D would also play a role. Vitamin D helps the bones absorb calcium and hold onto minerals. The higher a bone's mineral content, the stronger it is.

Rheumatoid arthritis and lupus patients also have been found to lack vitamin B12. A 2004 study published in *Rheumatology International* found that anemia and serum vitamin B12 deficiencies were much higher in patients suffering from rheumatoid arthritis, psoriatic arthritis, and systemic lupus erythematosus (Segal, 2004).

There are other factors involved in osteoporosis and rheumatoid arthritis as well, which we will be discussing in the sections on homocysteine and tumor necrosis factor.

Rosacea and Pancreatic Enzymes

Research done in Verona, Italy, showed a decrease in the pancreatic enzyme lipase. In the rosacea patients tested, lipase levels ranged from 18.5% to 66% of normal value (Barba, 1982). By providing a rich source of enzymes and beneficial bacteria, I believe the diet proposed in the last section of this book will eliminate rosacea, just as it did for my lupus rash. The following information points to a direct link between rosacea and pancreatic protease.

An article in *U.S. News & World Report* titled "A New Front in the Fight Against Rosacea," discussed findings that Rosacea was associated with abnormal proteins (MSNBC, 2007). Following is an excerpt of the article.

"In a study published in the online edition of Nature Medicine, research is pointing the way to potentially better therapy for rosacea. We spoke with its author, dermatologist Richard Gallo of the University of California-San Diego. Dr. Gallo stated, 'In rosacea, PEPTIDES are made abnormally. One hundred percent of the rosacea patients we looked at made more antimicrobial peptides than normal. And the peptides were processed into an ABNORMAL form that we found only in rosacea patient's skin, not in normal skin. This abnormal form triggers the body's inflammatory immune system, which normally activates when you have a cut or an injury.'" *Imagine this same response occurring 'inside' your body when it encounters a 'foreign' protein.*

This is huge. Here's where peptides come from; dietary proteins are broken down by proteases into amino acids and into peptides (short chains of amino acids). The connection is obvious. How could your body possibly form normal peptides from improperly broken down proteins and missing amino acids? In addition, this clearly shows what happens when the body encounters a protein that is not quite right, as we have observed in lupus.

Rosacea can also affect the eyes. One of the earliest manifestations of ocular rosacea may be blepharitis. Blepharitis refers to chronic inflammation of the eyelids. Eyelids become red and swollen and may develop scales and crusting. Other symptoms include: burning, itching, and a feeling of sand or grit in the eye. Blepharitis can occur even without cutaneous manifestations of rosacea present.

Blepharitis is another condition I suffered with myself. It was resolved quickly and completely when I began eating foods that replaced my missing pancreatic enzymes.

Type 2 Diabetes

Type 2 diabetes is a condition in which the pancreas no longer produces enough insulin, or when cells stop responding to insulin. When this happens, glucose in the blood can no longer be absorbed into the cells of the body. So, where does your body get insulin? The body needs to make it. It produces insulin from amino acids found in the foods we eat that contain protein; including meat, fish, dairy, and eggs. In order for the body to have access to the amino acids it needs to create insulin, pancreatic enzymes (proteases) must first break down the protein into individual amino acids for the body's use. Should the body become depleted of its reserve of any of the essential amino acids, it would no longer be able to produce insulin. *This is true if even one essential amino acid is missing.*

In patients with diabetes, the B12 connection has been established by researchers at the prestigious Warwick Medical School, University of Warwick. The University of Warwick researchers, led by Professor Paul Thornalley, have shown conclusively that diabetic patients are thiamine (B1) deficient in blood plasma. In a paper entitled "High prevalence of low plasma thiamine concentration in diabetes linked to a marker of vascular disease" published in *Diabetologia*, the team found *that thiamine concentration in blood plasma was decreased 76% in type 1 diabetic patients and 75% in type 2 diabetic patients.*

The paper states, "The researchers found that the decreased plasma thiamine concentration in clinical diabetes was not due to a deficiency of dietary input of thiamine. Rather it was due to a profound increased rate of removal of thiamine from the blood into the urine," (Thornalley, 2007). As we discussed earlier, if you are deficient in B12, you will not be able to absorb B1. It will be excreted in your urine.

One of the most common and troublesome complications of diabetes is diabetic autonomic neuropathy. According to the American Diabetes Association, "Autonomic neuropathy affects the autonomic nerves which control the bladder, intestinal tract, and the genitals, among other organs. Paralysis of the bladder is a common symptom. The nerves of the bladder no longer respond normally to pressure as the bladder fills with urine. As a result, urine stays in the bladder, which leads to urinary tract infections. Autonomic neuropathy can also cause erectile dysfunction when it affects the nerves that control erection. Diarrhea can occur when the nerves that control the small intestine are damaged. Constipation is another common result of damage to nerves in the intestines. Sometimes, the stomach is affected. It loses the ability to move food through the digestive system, causing vomiting and bloating," (American Diabetes Association, 2011).

In the prior discussion on dysautonomia (dysfunction of the autonomic nervous system) in fibromyalgia, we demonstrated the connection between dysautonomia and B12 deficiency. In the previous study entitled "Autonomic dysfunction and hemodynamics in vitamin B12 deficiency" researchers stated, "The results suggest that vitamin B12 deficiency causes autonomic dysfunction with similar hemodynamic consequences and patterns of autonomic failure as seen in diabetic autonomic neuropathy," (Beitzke, 2002).

Just as in rosacea, researchers have recently identified an abnormal peptide in patients with diabetes. Researchers at National Jewish Health and the University of Colorado Anschutz Medical Campus have identified the precise peptide that can trigger diabetes in mice. The findings support "An emerging theory about the origins of autoimmunity," as stated in an article from ScienceDaily. Following is an excerpt from the article that discusses this discovery.

"'Our findings contradict conventional wisdom, which suggests that insulin peptides that are well presented to the immune system trigger diabetes,' said John Kappler, Ph.D., Professor of Immunology at National Jewish Health. 'We believe, however, that the peptide we identified triggers diabetes precisely because it is so poorly presented to the immune system.' These findings support a theory recently posited by Kappler, Eisenbarth, and Brian Stadinski, Ph.D., of Harvard Medical School. They believe that, 'Poorly presented peptides are more likely to cause diabetes and other autoimmune diseases. This is the third time that a specific peptide and its binding register have been associated with autoimmune disease,' said Kappler. 'These findings have a direct link to human disease,'" (National Jewish Health, 2010).

Let's review what we've just read. Patients with diabetes are profoundly deficient in B1, which is directly connected to a lack of B12. In addition, prominent researchers have identified an 'abnormal peptide' in diabetes and believe that 'contrary to conventional wisdom' this abnormal peptide is triggering an immune response. Insulin is made in the pancreas from amino acids that come directly from dietary protein, and you cannot make insulin if even one amino acid is missing. Finally, diabetic autonomic neuropathy has the same pattern of autonomic failure as seen in autonomic dysfunction that is caused by vitamin B12 deficiency.

Given these facts, we have a great deal of evidence to support what we believe is the cause of diabetes.

The Diabetes Capital of the World

You may be surprised to learn that the country with the most vegetarians in the world also has the highest number of diabetics. The *International Journal of Diabetes in Developing Countries* calls India "the diabetes capital of the world." Ninety-five percent of the diabetics in India have type 2 diabetes.

The following study done in India and published in *Diabetologia*, concludes, "Vitamin B12 deficiency may be an important factor underlying the high risk of 'diabesity' in south Asian Indians." The lead researcher, Dr. Yajnik stated, "Multigenerational vegetarianism means that vitamin B12 deficiency is common in Indians...." In India, diabetes and other autoimmune diseases are caused primarily by a lack of B12 in the diet. This deficiency is not because they are unable to break down proteins and metabolize B12; however, the consequences are the same.

Once again, the criterion for a B12 deficiency was established at a very low level, 150 pg/mL. Even at that level, 43% were found deficient.

Low Plasma Vitamin B12 in Pregnancy is Associated with Gestational 'diabesity' and Later Diabetes

Krishnaveni, G.V., J.C. Hill, S.R. Veena, D.S. Bhat, A.K. Wills, C.L. Karat, C.S. Yajnik, C.H. Fall. 2009. *Diabetologia* 52 (11):2350-8.

Aims/Hypothesis: This study was designed to test the hypothesis that low plasma vitamin B(12) concentrations combined with high folate concentrations in pregnancy are associated with a higher incidence of gestational diabetes (GDM) and later diabetes.

Methods: Women (N = 785) attending the antenatal clinics of one hospital in Mysore, India, had their anthropometry, insulin resistance (homeostasis model assessment-2) and glucose tolerance assessed at 30 weeks' gestation (100 g oral glucose tolerance test; Carpenter-Coustan criteria) and at 5 years after delivery (75 g OGTT; WHO, 1999). Gestational vitamin B(12) and folate concentrations were measured in stored plasma samples.

Results: Low vitamin B(12) concentrations (<150 pmol/l, B(12) deficiency) were observed in 43% of women and low folate concentrations (<7 nmol/l) in 4%. B(12)-deficient women had higher body mass index (p < 0.001), sum of skinfold thickness (p < 0.001), insulin resistance (p = 0.02) and a higher incidence of GDM (8.7% vs 4.6%; OR 2.1, p = 0.02; p = 0.1 after adjusting for BMI) than non-deficient women. Among B(12)-deficient women, the incidence of GDM increased with folate concentration (5.4%, 10.5%, 10.9% from lowest to highest tertile, p = 0.04; p for interaction = 0.2). Vitamin B(12) deficiency during pregnancy was positively associated with skinfold thickness, insulin resistance (p < 0.05) and diabetes prevalence at 5 year follow-up (p = 0.009; p = 0.008 after adjusting for BMI). The association with diabetes became non-significant after excluding women with previous GDM (p = 0.06).

Conclusion: Maternal vitamin B(12) deficiency is associated with increased adiposity and, in turn, with insulin resistance and GDM. Vitamin B(12) deficiency may be an important factor underlying the high risk of 'diabesity' in south Asian Indians.

Myasthenia Gravis

The family of autoimmune diseases all share a direct ancestor. We have identified that ancestor, and tracing the family tree back to its roots will not be difficult now. Another direct link was found in the disease myasthenia gravis.

- Myasthenia: from the Greek words myelos (meaning muscle), and asthenia (meaning weakness)
- Gravis: from the Latin word, *gravidus* (meaning heavy or serious)

There were times we had to do a little digging to establish the connection of an autoimmune disease to missing enzymes. Not this time. Myasthenia gravis is caused, in part, by a lack of acetylcholine. *Vitamin B12 and folate are required for the synthesis of choline before becoming acetylcholine.*

During WWII, the development of myasthenia gravis in prisoners of war in Singapore was attributed to malnutrition. It is reported that a nutritious diet, with high vitamin content and plenty of liver, soon restored these prisoners to normal. Excess B12 is stored in our livers, so liver is one of the foods that contain the highest levels of B12. The fact that they recovered by eating liver shows they were able to properly digest the protein and simply lacked B12. In autoimmune disease, however, eating a lot of liver that you are not able to properly digest would just exacerbate the illness.

In myasthenia gravis, there is a problem in the transmission of nerve signals to your muscles. Normally, nerve endings release acetylcholine that attaches to receptors on your muscles. This signal tells your muscle to contract. Myasthenia gravis is considered an autoimmune disease because the body is producing antibodies that block the acetylcholine from attaching to receptors. One of the treatments for myasthenia gravis is removal of the thymus gland. An excerpt from an article in *ScienceDaily* talks about this treatment:

"Scientists have discovered that autoimmunity can be triggered in the thymus, where the immune system's T cells develop, if *T cells fail to recognize just one of the body's thousands of proteins as 'self.'* The research confirms an emerging view that autoimmunity can start in this cradle of the immune system, and not only at the sites where autoimmune diseases emerge, such as the pancreas in the case of type 1 diabetes or in the joints in rheumatoid arthritis. This single failure can lead to autoimmune disease," (University of California, 2006). This is what we have been emphasizing throughout this book. Proteins that are not properly broken down are not recognized by the body, and that will lead to autoimmune disease.

Abnormal Proteins Associated With CFIDS, Fibromyalgia, and Other Autoimmune Diseases

Spinal Tap Studies Discover Abnormal Proteins: These Don't Lie

In spinal tap studies conducted at the Georgetown University Proteomics Laboratory, Division of Rheumatology, Immunology & Allergy, researchers concluded, "This pilot study detected an *identical* set of central nervous system, innate immune and amyloidogenic proteins in cerebrospinal fluids from two independent cohorts of subjects with overlapping CFS, PGI (Persian Gulf War Illness), and fibromyalgia. Although syndrome names and definitions were different, the proteome and presumed pathological mechanisms may be shared," (Baraniuk, 2005).

The fact that researchers discovered an identical abnormal protein pattern in the spinal fluid of CFS, PGI, and fibromyalgia patients is quite significant. Spinal fluid studies use very advanced technology; therefore, the results are extremely definitive. The researchers also concluded that even though the names of these diseases were different, "the proteome and presumed pathological mechanisms may be shared." In other words, they all may originate from the same source.

The fact that abnormal proteins were discovered is also rather significant. They found abnormal proteins, rather than a virus or bacteria.

On Feb. 23, 2011, the *Wall Street Journal* reported on the results of another spinal fluid study done at the University of Medicine and Dentistry of New Jersey – New Jersey Medical School (Dockser-Marcus, 2011). It stated, "The researchers identified 738 proteins found in chronic fatigue patients, *but not healthy people or the treated Lyme patients.*"

The *Wall Street Journal* further reported, "Schutzer (lead researcher) is also involved in a separate study looking for microbes—including the virus XMRV—in the spinal fluid of 43 CFS patients. An abstract published earlier this month in *Annals of Neurology* reported that the team was unable to find XMRV in the spinal fluid of the CFS patients." *These findings show conclusively that there is an abnormal protein finding, as opposed to a viral, bacterial, or genetic finding.*

"They looked at a really important fluid, using a really advanced technology, and they found clear differences," said Suzanne Vernon, the scientific director of the Chronic Fatigue and Immune Dysfunction Syndrome Association of America. I'm very excited about this—you can't dispute these biological findings."

These proteins consisted of the following (Johnson, 2010):

- Two proteins suggesting a protease–antiprotease imbalance is present.
- Several proteins suggesting small amounts of bleeding in the brain could be caused by the aggregation of proteins (amyloids) in the blood vessel.
- An additional protein suggests increased free radical production is present.
- Another suggests problems with the vasoconstriction of the blood vessels and damage to the cells lining the blood vessels (the endothelial cells).
- An alternate protein suggesting altered rates of cell suicide (apoptosis) is present.

We can account for each and every one of these protein findings.

Notice the first protein finding, "protease-antiprotease imbalance is present." Remember, it was a lack of proteases and DNase 1 that caused the body to produce the protein NETs in lupus patients. This also led to the body's inability to break them down. Now we find a lack of proteases in the spinal fluid of fibromyalgia and chronic fatigue syndrome patients as well.

Amyloid proteins are revealed in the second finding and appear to be key elements of the protein signature. Amyloid proteins are peptides that get folded improperly as they are being made. Proteins trigger cellular activity by locking into each other like three dimensional keys. Since shape in a protein is everything, improper folding can cause a protein to be useless or even dangerous. These amyloid proteins are made in the body from amino acids. You will not be able to produce normal proteins if you are missing amino acids. Amino acids are derived from dietary proteins. If you are lacking the pancreatic enzymes (proteases) that are responsible for breaking down dietary protein into amino acids, you will not be able to produce normally-shaped proteins, but rather misshapen amyloids. Your immune system will then mount an immune response to them, because they are not recognized by your body. Your body is not attacking you, it is attacking abnormal proteins.

The same amyloids that have now been identified in chronic fatigue syndrome and fibromyalgia also exist in lupus, multiple sclerosis, rheumatoid arthritis, and Sjögren's. This is called secondary amyloidosis. There is also a disease called primary amyloidosis. According to Mayo Clinic, these amyloids can build up in the heart, kidney, liver, spleen, nerves, skin, blood vessels, and gastrointestinal tract. Here are some of the symptoms—irregular heartbeats, numbness, shortness of breath, swelling, and weak grip. It can also lead to endocrine failure, as well as heart, kidney, and respiratory failure. These diseases all share many of the same symptoms because they have the same abnormal proteins or amyloids. These diseases also share the same cause, which is the creation of amyloids instead of properly folded proteins, because the body lacks amino acids.

In the last three protein findings, we see increased free radical production, problems with vasoconstriction of the blood vessels, damage to the cells lining the blood vessels (the endothelial cells), and cell suicide or apoptosis. We will thoroughly address these findings in the next section.

Chapter 2 THE DISCOVERY

Homocysteine

In this section, we will be introducing a new player to the autoimmune disease process. We will focus on the vascular components of autoimmune disease, such as Raynaud's, migraines, and increased risk of heart disease and stroke. The new player's name is "homocysteine." If you suffer with Raynaud's, migraines, or heart disease, you have likely just found out why.

Like cholesterol, homocysteine performs a desirable function. It is derived from the essential amino acid methionine and is used to build and maintain tissue. During normal conditions, excess homocysteine, with the help of B12, is converted back to methionine or broken down for excretion. The problem arises when the conversion process fails due to the lack of B12. Homocysteine and B12 are so closely connected, that currently, one of the most accurate tests for B12 deficiency is to check for elevated homocysteine levels. If B12 is deficient, homocysteine goes up. *Way up.*

An increased serum concentration of homocysteine is now recognized as a major risk factor in heart disease and stroke. Researchers at Johns Hopkins Medical Institutions found that lupus (SLE) patients have an increased risk of suffering strokes, heart attacks, and other arterial thrombotic events, such as gangrene of the fingers (Petri, 1996). They attributed this higher risk, at least partially, to a greater propensity among SLE patients to develop premature atherosclerosis due to a lack of B12, and the subsequent rise in homocysteine. High concentrations of homocysteine have previously been linked to an increased risk of stroke and coronary artery disease. Many SLE patients have high homocysteine levels. The researchers concluded, "SLE patients with elevated homocysteine levels have a 2.4 times higher risk of having a stroke and a 3.5 times higher risk of having an arterial thrombotic event."

Increased homocysteine levels contribute to atherosclerosis in the following ways:

- Oxidation of LDL (low-density lipoprotein) cholesterol, making it more likely to stick to injured vessels
- Induces oxidative stress and impairs the ability of blood vessels to expand and contract
- Increases blood clot formation
- Injures the lining of blood vessel walls
- Accelerates smooth muscle growth, contributing to the narrowing of blood vessel walls

The following study from the Jean Mayer USDA Human Nutrition Research Center on Aging followed 1,947 participants over a period of 9.9 years in order to determine whether homocysteine levels predicted stroke incidence in elderly persons (Bostom, 1999). The researchers concluded that, "Nonfasting total homocysteine levels are an independent risk factor for incident stroke in elderly persons."

Nonfasting Plasma Total Homocysteine Levels and Stroke Incidence in Elderly Persons: The Framingham Study

Bostom, A.G., I.H. Rosenberg, H. Silbershatz, P.F. Jaques, J. Selhub, R.B. D'Agostino, P.W. Wilson, P.A. Wolf. 1999. Ann Intern Med 131(5):325-5.

Background: Total homocysteine levels are associated with arteriosclerotic outcomes.

Objective: To determine whether total homocysteine levels predict incident stroke in elderly persons.

Design: Prospective population-based cohort study with 9.9 years of follow-up.

Setting: Framingham, Massachusetts.

Patients: 1947 Framingham Study participants (1158 women and 789 men; mean age +/- SD, 70 +/- 7 years).

Measurements: Baseline total homocysteine levels and 9.9-year stroke incidence.

Results: The quartiles of nonfasting total homocysteine levels were as follows: quartile 1, 4.13 to 9.25 micromol/L; quartile 2, 9.26 to 11.43 micromol/L; quartile 3, 11.44 to 14.23 micromol/L; quartile 4, 14.24 to 219.84 micromol/L. During follow-up, 165 incident strokes occurred. In proportional hazards models adjusted for age, sex, systolic blood pressure, diabetes, smoking, and history of atrial fibrillation and coronary heart disease, relative risk (RR) estimates comparing quartile 1 with the other three quartiles were as follows: quartile 2 compared with quartile 1--RR, 1.32 (95% CI, 0.81 to 2.14); quartile 3 compared with quartile 1--RR, 1.44 (CI, 0.89 to 2.34); quartile 4 compared with quartile 1--RR, 1.82 (CI, 1.14 to 2.91). The linear trend across the quartiles was significant ($P < 0.001$).

Conclusion: Nonfasting total homocysteine levels are an independent risk factor for incident stroke in elderly persons

There is also evidence that homocysteine disrupts proper brain functioning. Homocysteine appears to inappropriately stimulate some nerve cell receptors, which can hinder normal brain function. High homocysteine levels can interfere with the synthesis of S-adenosylmethionine (SAMe) and lead to increased levels of S-adenosyl homocysteine. This may adversely affect a whole range of brain processes, and cause or worsen psychological abnormalities.

This next article, published in *ScienceDaily*, highlights the cerebral microvascular dysfunction associated with B12 deficiency and resulting high homocysteine levels.

B-Vitamin Deficiency May Cause Vascular Cognitive Impairment
ScienceDaily, Sep. 2, 2008

Researchers at the Jean Mayer USDA Human Nutrition Research Center on Aging (HNRCA) at Tufts University looked at Vitamin B deficiency, homocysteine levels and the effect on Vascular Cognitive Impairment. The researchers fed mice a diet deficient in three vitamins B12, folate, and B6. The deficiency caused cognitive dysfunction and reductions in brain capillary length and density in the mice.

Aron Troen, PhD, the study's lead author explains, "Mice fed a diet deficient in folate and vitamins B12 and B6 demonstrated significant deficits in spatial learning and memory compared with normal mice."

Troen goes on to say, "based on the findings of our study, we theorize that a deficiency of B-vitamins induces a metabolic disorder that manifests with high homocysteine, as well as cerebral microvascular dysfunction".

Journal Reference:

Troen et al. 2008. B-vitamin deficiency causes hyperhomocysteinemia and vascular cognitive impairment in mice. Proceedings of the *Proceedings of the National Academy of Sciences* 105(34):12474.

In the following cross-sectional study, researchers from Rush University Medical Center in Chicago state, "Homocysteine concentrations were associated with decreased brain volume," (Tangney, 2011). Over nearly five years of follow-up, markers of B12 insufficiency also predicted lower global cognitive scores. The researchers concluded that, "Vitamin B12 may affect the brain through multiple mechanisms."

Vitamin B12, Cognition, and Brain MRI Measures: A Cross-Sectional Examination

Tangney, C.C., N.T. Aggarwal, H. Li, R.S. Wilson, C. Decarli, D.A. Evans, M.C. Morris. 2011. *Neurology* 77(13):1276-82.

Objective: To investigate the interrelations of serum vitamin B12 markers with brain volumes, cerebral infarcts, and performance in different cognitive domains in a biracial population sample cross-sectionally.

Methods: In 121 community-dwelling participants of the Chicago Health and Aging Project, serum markers of vitamin B12 status were related to summary measures of neuropsychological tests of 5 cognitive domains and brain MRI measures obtained on average 4.6 years later among 121 older adults.

Results: Concentrations of all vitamin B12-related markers, but not serum vitamin B12 itself, were associated with global cognitive function and with total brain volume. Methylmalonate levels were associated with poorer episodic memory and perceptual speed, and cystathionine and 2-methylcitrate with poorer episodic and semantic memory. Homocysteine concentrations were associated with decreased total brain volume. The homocysteine-global cognition effect was modified and no longer statistically significant with adjustment for white matter volume or cerebral infarcts. The methylmalonate-global cognition effect was modified and no longer significant with adjustment for total brain volume.

Conclusions: Methylmalonate, a specific marker of B12 deficiency, may affect cognition by reducing total brain volume whereas the effect of homocysteine (nonspecific to vitamin B12 deficiency) on cognitive performance may be mediated through increased white matter hyperintensity and cerebral infarcts. Vitamin B12 status may affect the brain through multiple mechanisms.

The following study from Oxford University, found that older people with lower than average vitamin B12 levels were six times more likely to experience brain shrinkage (Vogiatzoglou, 2008). The study, published in *Neurology*, tested 107 volunteers who had no mental impairments. Researchers used MRI scans to measure brain volume and blood tests to record vitamin B12 levels. They divided the subjects into three groups, based on their level of the vitamin, and followed them for five years. The decrease in brain volume was greater among those with lower vitamin B12 and higher plasma levels at baseline. An article in The New York Times discusses this study, saying that, "Failure to properly absorb vitamin B12, found in meat, milk and eggs, has been implicated in various neurological disorders. Now a British study suggests that low levels of the vitamin in older people may cause the brain to shrink," (Bakalar, 2008).

Vitamin B12 Status and Rate of Brain Volume Loss in Community-Dwelling Elderly

Vogiatzoglou, A, H. Refsum, C. Johnston, S.M. Smith, K.M. Bradley, C. de Jager, M.M. Budge, A.D. Smith. 2008. Neurology 71(11):826-32.

Objectives: To investigate the relationship between markers of vitamin B(12) status and brain volume loss per year over a 5-year period in an elderly population.

Methods: A prospective study of 107 community-dwelling volunteers aged 61 to 87 years without cognitive impairment at enrollment. Volunteers were assessed yearly by clinical examination, MRI scans, and cognitive tests. Blood was collected at baseline for measurement of plasma vitamin B(12), transcobalamin (TC), holotranscobalamin (holoTC), methylmalonic acid (MMA), total homocysteine (tHcy), and serum folate.

Results: The decrease in brain volume was greater among those with lower vitamin B(12) and holoTC levels and higher plasma tHcy and MMA levels at baseline. Linear regression analysis showed that associations with vitamin B(12) and holoTC remained significant after adjustment for age, sex, creatinine, education, initial brain volume, cognitive test scores, systolic blood pressure, ApoE epsilon4 status, tHcy, and folate. Using the upper (for the vitamins) or lower tertile (for the metabolites) as reference in logistic regression analysis and adjusting for the above covariates, vitamin B(12) in the bottom tertile (<308 pmol/L) was associated with increased rate of brain volume loss (odds ratio 6.17, 95% CI 1.25-30.47). The association was similar for low levels of holoTC (<54 pmol/L) (odds ratio 5.99, 95% CI 1.21-29.81) and for low TC saturation. High levels of MMA or tHcy or low levels of folate were not associated with brain volume loss.

Conclusion: Low vitamin B(12) status should be further investigated as a modifiable cause of brain atrophy and of likely subsequent cognitive impairment in the elderly.

Numerous studies are finding evidence that low B12 and high homocysteine are related to the risk of developing Alzheimer's. Researchers from the University of California-Davis Medical Center found homocysteine was "significantly higher" in patients with Alzheimer's (Miller, 1999).

Homocysteine and Alzheimer's Disease
Miller, J.W. 1999. Nutr Rev 57(4):126-9.

Abstract: In a recent case-control study of 164 patients with clinically diagnosed Alzheimer's disease (AD), including 76 patients with the AD diagnosis confirmed postmortem, mean total serum homocysteine concentration was found to be significantly higher than that of a control group of elderly individuals with no evidence of cognitive impairment. Because homocysteine is considered an independent risk factor for vascular disease, this finding is consistent with the emerging hypothesis that vascular disease is a contributing factor in the pathogenesis of AD.

The following study, published in Neurology, found that those with the highest levels of B12 were the least likely to be diagnosed with dementia (Hooshmand, 2010). The authors followed 271 Finnish people (ages 65 to 79) for 7 years, none of whom had previously presented any symptoms of Alzheimer's disease. Interestingly, 17 of the subjects ended-up developing

Alzheimer's disease during the course of the study, and the researchers found that with each micromolar increase in blood homocysteine level, the risk of Alzheimer's disease increased by 16%. Professor Helga Refsum, from the University of Oslo, stated the study was "futher evidence" that low levels of B12 were linked to Alzheimer's.

Homocysteine and Holotranscobalamin and the Risk of Alzheimer Disease: A Longitudinal Study
Hooshmand B, Solomon A, Kåreholt I, Leiviskä J, Rusanen M, Ahtiluoto S, Winblad B, Laatikainen T, Soininen H, Kivipelto M. 2010. Neurology 75(16):1408-14.

Objective: To examine the relation between serum levels of homocysteine (tHcy) and holotranscobalamin (holoTC), the active fraction of vitamin B12, and risk of incident Alzheimer disease (AD) in a sample of Finnish community-dwelling elderly.

Conclusions: This study suggests that both tHcy and holoTC may be involved in the development of AD. The tHcy-AD link may be partly explained by serum holoTC. The role of holoTC in AD should be further investigated.

How Dangerous is Homocysteine?

Homocysteine has been found to be approximately *40 times more predictive* than cholesterol in assessing risk of cardiovascular disease. "An avalanche of new studies suggests that an amino acid called homocysteine plays a critical role in destroying our arteries," (Newsweek, 1997).

A study conducted at Brigham and Women's Hospital and Harvard Medical School in Boston, Massachusetts, followed 14,915 doctors. The study revealed that participants with high homocysteine levels had 3.4 times greater risk of heart attack than doctors with lower homocysteine levels (Stampfer, 1992). That's 340%! Homocysteine is a potent nerve and blood vessel toxin. We will now look at its role in Raynaud's, fibromyalgia, chronic fatigue syndrome, rheumatoid arthritis, COPD, scleroderma, diabetic neuropathy, migraines, multiple sclerosis, heart disease, connective-tissue disease, hypothyroidism, vision complications, and even cancer.

Here are two studies that link homocysteine to Raynaud's.

Elevated Homocysteine Levels in Patients with Raynaud's Syndrome

Levy, Y., J. George, P. Langevitz, D. Harats, R. Doolman, B.A. Sela, Y. Shoenfield. 1999. *Journal of Rheumatology* 26:2383-85.

Raynaud's phenomenon (RP) involves a disruption of blood flow to fingers or toes resulting in cold, numbness, and a characteristic white colour of the affected parts. RP is often associated with scleroderma or systemic lupus erythematosus (secondary RP), but can also occur as a separate disease entity (primary RP or Raynaud's disease). The cause of the phenomenon is unknown, but it is believed that an abnormality in the endothelium (the single layer of cells that line the blood vessels) is involved.

Now researchers at Tel-Aviv University report that high blood plasma levels of homocysteine are closely associated with RP. Their study involved 10 patients with primary RP, 10 patients with RP secondary to scleroderma, and 20 healthy controls. The researchers measured plasma levels of homocysteine and folate (folic acid) in fasting blood samples taken from all participants. They found the average (mean) homocysteine level of controls to be 5.9 micromol/L; patients with primary RP had a mean homocysteine level of 15.5 micromol/L while patients with secondary RP had a mean level of 11.6 micromol/L. A level above 10.5 micromol/L is considered excessive and is associated with an increased risk for heart disease and stroke. Homocysteine levels tend to be inversely proportional to folate levels. In this study controls had a mean folate level of 8.84 nanograms/mL, patients with primary RP had a mean level of only 4.79 ng/mL while patients with secondary RP had a mean level of 7.15 ng/mL.

The researchers speculate that high homocysteine levels may be, at least in part, responsible for the abnormal behaviour of the endothelium in RP patients. They suggest further work to investigate this connection and, if indeed proven, recommend that RP patients be treated with folic acid supplementation.

Homocysteine and Raynaud's Phenomenon: A Review

Lazzerini, P.E., P.L. Capecchi, S. Bisogno, M. Cozzalupi, P.C. Rossi, F.L. Pasini. 2010. *Autoimmun Rev* 9(3):181-7.

Raynaud's phenomenon, categorized as primary and secondary when occurring isolated or in association with an underlying disease, respectively, is a paroxysmal and recurrent acral ischemia resulting from an abnormal arterial vasospastic response to cold or emotional stress. The key issue in the pathogenesis of Raynaud's phenomenon is presumed to be a dysregulation in the mechanisms of vascular motility resulting in an imbalance between vasodilatation and vasoconstriction. Homocysteine, a non-protein forming sulphured amino acid proposed as an independent risk factor for atherothrombosis in the general population, clearly demonstrated to produce vascular damage through mechanisms also including endothelial injury and modifications in circulating mediators of vasomotion. The rationale for homocysteine involvement in the pathogenesis of Raynaud's phenomenon led some authors to investigate the possible association between mild hyperhomocysteinemia and such a vascular disturbance, particularly in the course of connective tissue disease. Here we review data regarding this putative association and the supposed mechanisms involved, also discussing the emblematic case of a patient with new-onset severe Raynaud's phenomenon and markedly elevated homocysteinemia.

A study published in the *Scandinavian Journal of Rheumatology* links fibromyalgia and chronic fatigue syndrome to low vitamin B12 and high homocysteine in cerebrospinal fluid (Regland, 1997). Here is the conclusion from the study, "This study provides convincing preliminary evidence that a high homocysteine level in cerebrospinal fluid is an underlying factor in patients suffering from fibromyalgia and chronic fatigue syndrome. Low vitamin B12 levels in cerebrospinal fluid and possibly low SAMe levels are implicated as contributing factors. Additional evidence from other studies further support the idea that deficiencies in enzymatic pathways in the brain involving vitamin B12, homocysteine, and folic acid underlie a range of neurological disorders. Deficiencies in these essential biochemical pathways in the brain should be considered by health practitioners in the evaluation of successful interventions for reversing symptoms of fibromyalgia, chronic fatigue syndrome, and other neurological conditions."

Wow! Someone in Sweden sure got it right.

Rheumatoid Arthritis and Homocysteine

Statistics for patients with rheumatoid arthritis are equally grim. One-third to one-half of premature deaths in rheumatoid arthritis are due to cardiovascular disease. A study published in the December 15, 2008 issue of *Arthritis and Rheumatism* found there was a 50% increased risk of death from ischemic heart disease and stroke in rheumatoid arthritis patients compared to the general population (Aviña-Zubieta, 2008).

Homocysteine causes superoxide radicals to form in the blood, which kill cells in the blood vessel walls. Once damaged, the affected area swells and forms a 'rough spot' where sticky cholesterol, along with platelets and white blood cells that arrive to fix the damage, start to collect plaque, thus contributing to these grim statistics.

A study published in the *Journal of Internal Medicine* looked at the risk of ischemic heart disease associated with rheumatoid arthritis and found, "The risk of having a heart attack is 60% higher just a year after a patient has been diagnosed with rheumatoid arthritis…," (Wiley-Blackwell, 2010).

The following study abstract shows the relationship between patients with rheumatoid arthritis and increased levels of homocysteine. This leads to increased mortality related to cardiovascular disease.

Abnormal Homocysteine Metabolism in Rheumatoid Arthritis

Roubenoff, R., P. Dellaripa, M.R. Nadeau, L.W. Abad, B.A. Muldoon, J. Selhub, I.H. Rosenberg IH. 1997. *Arthritis Rheum.* 40(4):718-22.

Objective: Assess total homocysteine (tHcy) metabolism in patients with rheumatoid arthritis (RA).

Methods: Assessments were performed to determine the fasting levels of tHcy and the increase in tHcy in response to methionine (Met) challenge in blood samples from 28 patients with RA and 20 healthy age-matched control subjects.

Results: Fasting levels of tHcy were 33% higher in the RA patients than in the control subjects (mean +/- SD 11.7 +/- 1.5 nmoles/ml versus 8.8 +/- 1.1 nmoles/ml; $P < 0.01$). Four hours after Met challenge, the increase in plasma tHcy levels (delta tHcy) was higher in the RA patients (20.9 +/- 10.4 nmoles/ml) than in the control subjects (15.5 +/- 1.6 nmoles/ml) ($P < 0.02$). In a subgroup analysis, the delta tHcy in patients taking methotrexate (12.9 +/- 2.2 nmoles/ml) did not differ from that in the control group, while the delta tHcy in patients not taking methotrexate (25.3 +/- 1.7 nmoles/ml) was significantly higher ($P < 0.0001$).

Conclusion: Elevated tHcy levels occur commonly in patients with RA, and may explain some of the increased cardiovascular mortality seen in such patients. Studies of the prevalence and mechanism of hyperhomocysteinemia in RA are warranted.

COPD, Rheumatoid Arthritis, and Homocysteine

COPD, or chronic obstructive pulmonary disease, is a progressive disease that makes it hard to breathe. COPD can cause coughing that produces large amounts of mucus, wheezing, shortness of breath, and chest tightness, among other symptoms. In COPD, the small capillaries that run through the walls of the air sacs in the lungs are damaged or completely destroyed. More than 12 million people are currently diagnosed with COPD. It is the fourth leading cause of death in the United States.

Now, a new study presented at the EULAR 2011 Annual Congress (European League Against Rheumatism) has confirmed a link between rheumatoid arthritis and COPD. An article on this study in *News-Medical* states, "Patients with rheumatoid arthritis are two times more likely to have COPD than healthy controls. The study of 15,766 patients with RA and 15,340 controls found that the prevalence of COPD was significantly higher in RA patients than healthy controls. Interestingly, the link was still significant after risk factors common in both RA and COPD patients, such as smoking, obesity and socioeconomic status, were controlled for," (News-Medical, 2011). The large, population-based study was performed using the patient database of Israel's largest healthcare provider, Clalit Health Services.

The researchers concluded, "We know that similar changes in core physiological processes cause symptoms in RA and COPD....."

COPD and RA share a common link. This link would explain the "similar changes in core physiological processes" between RA and COPD. The link is homocysteine. The following study confirms this association.

Plasma Homocysteine is Elevated in COPD Patients and is Related to COPD Severity
Seemungal, T.A., J.C. Lun, G. Davis, C. Neblett, N. Chinyepi, C. Dookhan, S. Drakes, E. Mandeville, F. Nana, S. Sethake, C.P. King, L. PintoPereira, J. Delisle, T.M. Wilkenson, J.A. Wedzicha. 2007. *Int J Chron Obstruct Pulmon Dis* 2(3):313-21.

Background: Although recent studies have found that total plasma homocysteine (tHCY) and chronic obstructive pulmonary disease (COPD) are both risk factors for cardiac disease, there have been few studies of plasma homocysteine levels in COPD patients. We tested the hypothesis that total plasma homocysteine (tHCY) would be elevated in patients diagnosed with COPD compared with controls.

Methods: We studied 29 COPD outpatients and 25 asymptomatic subjects (controls) over age 55 years with measurement of forced expiratory volume in one second (FEV1), forced vital capacity (FVC), St. Georges Respiratory Questionnaire (SGRQ) score, tHCY and serum C-reactive protein (sCRP).

Results: There was no difference between controls vs. COPD patients in mean age or gender but mean (SD) FEV_1 was 2.25 (0.77) vs 1.43 (0.60) L; FEV_1% predicted 76.1 (17.2) vs 49.1 (16.3) $p < 0.001$ in both cases. Median (IQR) tHCY was 8.22 (6.63, 9.55) in controls vs 10.96 (7.56, 13.60) micromol/l for COPD, $p = 0.006$ and sCRP 0.89 (0.47, 2.55) vs 2.05 (0.86, 6.19) mg/l, $p = 0.023$. tHCY(log) was also higher in (r, p) smokers (0.448, 0.001), patients with low FEV_1% (−0.397, 0.003), males (0.475, <0.001), but high SGRQ Total score (0.289, 0.034), and high sCRP (0.316, 0.038). tHCY(log) was independently related to (regression coefficient, p) sCRP(log) (0.087, 0.024), male gender (0.345, <0.001) and presence of COPD (0.194, 0.031). Median (IQR) tHCY GOLD Stage I and II 8.05 (7.28, 11.04), GOLD Stage III and IV: 11.83(9.30, 18.30); p = 0.023.

Conclusions: Plasma homocysteine is significantly elevated in COPD patients relative to age and sex-matched controls and is related to serum CRP and COPD severity.

According to the Lupus Foundation of America, the lungs are frequently affected in people with lupus, as they are with many other autoimmune diseases, such as scleroderma. The following study from the *Journal of Rheumatology* states, "In patients with scleroderma the homocysteine concentration was significantly higher than in controls. We found a significant association between plasma homocysteine concentration and severity of lung involvement ..." The researchers believe that elevated homocysteine may worsen injury of the endothelium. They concluded, "Our data support the hypothesis that homocysteine could be involved in the pathogenetic process of scleroderma pulmonary lung involvement."

Homocysteine Plasma Concentration is Related to Severity of Lung Impairment in Scleroderma

Caramaschi, P., N. Martinelli, D. Biasi, A. Carletto, G. Faccini, A. Volpe, M. Ferrari, C. Scambi, L.M. Bambara. 2003. J Rheumatol 30(2):298-304.

Objective: To investigate the correlation between plasma concentration of total homocysteine and pulmonary involvement in patients with limited or diffuse scleroderma (systemic sclerosis, SSc).

Conclusion: High level of homocysteinemia is associated with an increased risk of pulmonary disease in patients with scleroderma. We hypothesize that hyperhomocysteinemia may worsen injury of the endothelium, a key lesion in scleroderma disease, favoring the development of lung involvement. "Our data support the hypothesis that homocysteine could be involved in the pathogenetic process of scleroderma pulmonary involvement". (J Rheumatol 2003;30:298-304).

Type 2 Diabetes and Homocysteine
Diabetic Neuropathy and Homocysteine

In the following study of 65 patients with type 2 diabetes, elevated levels of homocysteine were found to be independently associated with the prevalence of peripheral neuropathy. The authors suggested that this association could be explained either by direct cytotoxic effects on nerve function, or by small vessel occlusions caused by endothelial damage. This results in a loss of blood supply to nerve fibers, a pathogenetic mechanism of peripheral neuropathy.

Relation Between Homocysteinaemia and Diabetic Neuropathy in Patients with Type 2 Diabetes Mellitus

Ambrosch, A., J. Dierkes, R. Lobmann, W. Kühne, W. König, C. Luley, H. Lehnert. 2001. *Diabet Med.* 18(3):185-92.

Aims: Limited data are available on determinants of diabetic neuropathy as its pathogenesis is multifactorial. Since homocysteine exhibits toxic effects on vascular endothelial cells, the association between homocysteine and the prevalence of neuropathy in Type 2 diabetes mellitus was investigated.

Methods: A total of 65 Type 2 diabetic patients were consecutively enrolled into the study. Neuropathy was diagnosed according to clinical symptoms, clinical examination, electrophysiological sensory testing and autonomic function testing. With regard to homocysteine-related parameters, plasma homocysteine, folate, vitamin B12, vitamin B6 and renal function (creatinine, ceratinine clearance, cystatin C) were measured, and the C677T polymorphism of the methylenetetrahydrofolate reductase gene was determined.

Results: Forty-three of the Type 2 diabetic patients were classified as suffering from neuropathy. Both patient groups were comparable with regard to demographic data, blood pressure, glucose metabolism, renal function and homocysteine-related vitamins. In contrast, homocysteine levels (P = 0.04) and the frequency of hyperhomocysteinemia (>or= 15 micromol/l) (P = 0.01) were significantly increased in neuropathic patients. In a logistic regression model with neuropathy as dependent variable, homocysteine (adjusted for creatinine, homocysteine-related vitamins, HbA1c and duration of diabetes) was the only significant variable associated with the prevalence of neuropathy (odds ratio for homocysteine per 5 micromol/l increase: 2.60 (95% confidence interval 1.07-6.33)).

Conclusion: The data indicate that homocysteine is independently associated with the prevalence of diabetic neuropathy in a collective of Type 2 diabetic patients. A larger, prospective study would be desirable to clarify the role of homocysteine in the pathogenesis of diabetic neuropathy.

The following study, published in the *Annals of Internal Medicine*, concluded that, "In this large cohort of patients with type 2 diabetes, plasma homocysteine was a strong and independent risk factor for CHD (coronary heart disease) events," (Soinio, 2004).

Elevated Plasma Homocysteine Level Is an Independent Predictor of Coronary Heart Disease Events in Patients with Type 2 Diabetes Mellitus

Soinio, M., J. Marniemi, M. Laakso, S. Lehto, T. Rönnemaa. 2004. Ann Intern Med 140(2):94-100.

Background: High plasma homocysteine level has been associated with increased risk for coronary heart disease (CHD) events in nondiabetic individuals, especially in those with previously diagnosed CHD. In persons with type 2 diabetes mellitus, the association between homocysteine level and cardiovascular disease may be stronger than that in nondiabetic individuals, but no large prospective studies have examined the relationship between homocysteine level and CHD mortality in persons with type 2 diabetes.

Objective: To investigate whether moderately elevated plasma homocysteine levels are independently related to increased incidence of fatal and nonfatal CHD events in persons with type 2 diabetes.

Design: Prospective study.

Setting: Finnish sample of patients with type 2 diabetes.

Patients: 462 men and 368 women who were 45 to 64 years of age at baseline.

Measurements: Coronary heart disease mortality and incidence of nonfatal myocardial infarction during the 7-year follow-up.

Results: Participants with plasma homocysteine levels of 15 μmol/L or more at baseline had a higher risk for CHD death than those with plasma homocysteine levels less than 15 μmol/L (26.1% and 13.5%, respectively; P = 0.005). The risks for all CHD events were 36.2% and 22.6%, respectively (P = 0.011). In Cox regression analyses, elevated plasma homocysteine level was significantly associated with CHD mortality (P < 0.001) and all CHD events (P = 0.002) even after adjustment for confounding variables, including creatinine clearance. In participants without myocardial infarction at baseline, moderate hyperhomocysteinemia was also associated with CHD mortality and all CHD events in univariate (P < 0.001 and P = 0.006, respectively) and multivariate Cox regression analyses (P < 0.001 and P = 0.004, respectively).

Conclusions: In this large cohort of patients with type 2 diabetes, plasma homocysteine level was a strong and independent risk factor for CHD events.

Homocysteine is also associated with ulceration in type 2 diabetes. The study entitled "Plasma Homocysteine Levels are Associated with Ulceration of the Foot In Patients with Type 2 Diabetes" concluded that "for each micromol increase in plasma homocysteine levels there was a 10% increase in the risk of diabetic foot ulceration," (González, 2010).

Migraines and Homocysteine

Compared with the general population, people with lupus may be twice as likely to experience migraine headaches, commonly known as lupus headaches. The paper entitled "A study of headaches and migraine in Sjögren's syndrome and other rheumatic disorders" reported that nearly half (46%) of Sjögren's patients and 32% of patients with scleroderma suffer from migraines as well (Pal, 1989). It concluded that, "There was a significant association between occurrence of Raynaud's phenomenon and migraine. Small vessel pathology may underlie both migraine and Raynaud's phenomenon in these connective tissue disorders-as has been suggested in systemic lupus erythematosus."

In Headache: The Journal of Head and Face Pain, author Cris S. Constantinescu M.D., Ph.D., states, "Migraine and Raynaud phenomenon often coexist and may reflect similar vascular reactions. Both have been associated with vascular endothelial cell dysfunction," (Constantinescu, 2002).

The following study found that homocysteine levels were significantly higher in patients with migraine with aura (MA) than in healthy controls.

Homocysteine Plasma Levels in Patients With Migraine With Aura

Moschiano. F., D. D'Amico, S. Usai, L. Grazzi, M. Di Stefano, E. Ciusani, N. Erba, G. Bussone. 2008, *Neurol Sci* 29(Suppl. 1):S173-5.

Abstract: We investigated homocysteine plasma levels in 136 MA sufferers and in 117 sex-and age-matched controls. Mean homocysteine plasma levels - as well as the proportion of subjects with hyperhomocysteinaemia - were significantly higher in patients with MA than in healthy controls. Hyperhomocysteinaemia may be a link between MA and ischaemic stroke.

The next study, done in Japan, is notably and appropriately titled "Homocysteine Induces Programmed Cell Death in Human Vascular Endothelial Cells."

Homocysteine Induces Programmed Cell Death in Human Vascular Endothelial Cells Through Activation of the Unfolded Protein Response

Zhang, C, Y. Cai, M.T. Adachi, S. Oshiro, T. Aso, R.J. Kaufman, S. Kitajima. 2001. *J Biol Chem* 276(38):35867-74.

Severe hyperhomocysteinemia is associated with endothelial cell injury that may contribute to an increased incidence of thromboembolic disease. In this study, homocysteine induced programmed cell death in human umbilical vein endothelial cells as measured by TdT-mediated dUTP nick end labeling assay, DNA ladder formation, induction of caspase 3-like activity, and cleavage of procaspase 3. Homocysteine-induced cell death was specific to homocysteine, was not mediated by oxidative stress, and was mimicked by inducers of the unfolded protein response (UPR), a signal transduction pathway activated by the accumulation of unfolded proteins in the lumen of the endoplasmic reticulum. Dominant negative forms of the endoplasmic reticulum-resident protein kinases IRE1alpha and -beta, which function as signal transducers of the UPR, prevented the activation of glucose-regulated protein 78/immunoglobulin chain-binding protein and C/EBP homologous protein/growth arrest and DNA damage-inducible protein 153 in response to homocysteine. Furthermore, overexpression of the point mutants of IRE1 with defective RNase more effectively suppressed the cell death than the kinase-defective mutant. These results indicate that homocysteine induces apoptosis in human umbilical vein endothelial cells by activation of the UPR and is signaled through IRE1. The studies implicate that the UPR may cause endothelial cell injury associated with severe hyperhomocysteinemia.

The previous studies on Raynaud's and migraines, in addition to the study from Japan, show the damage homocysteine can do to the vascular endothelial cells. Endothelial cells line the entire circulatory system, from the heart to the smallest capillary. The following study from the University of Michigan highlights the increased risk of heart disease for lupus patients. The researchers concluded that something must be damaging the *endothelial cell layer* to cause the protective cells to commit "mass suicide."

U-M Study: High Heart Disease Risk for Lupus Patients May Be Linked to Rapid Death of Blood Vessel Lining Cells
Gavin, K., 11 November 2003.

Mass suicide by protective cells that line every blood vessel in the body may be to blame for the increased risk of heart and vascular disease faced by patients with the autoimmune disease known as lupus, new research suggests.

The new study suggests that lupus patients' heightened heart risk may be due to the rapid death and much-too-slow replacement of endothelial cells, which normally keep plaques and clots from forming in blood vessels. Loss of these cells through accelerated apoptosis may affect vascular and heart health in many ways, says Rajagopalan, since endothelial cells serve an important barrier function, and make nitric oxide that regulates blood vessel dilation and contraction and blood flow.

Rajagopalan and Kaplan, along with a team of U-M colleagues, suspected something must be damaging the endothelial cell layer in order to cause cardiovascular disease in women with no other risk factors besides lupus. They set out to determine if they could see these apoptotic endothelial cells in the blood, and correlate them to both vascular function and the flaring up of lupus symptoms.

"We hypothesized that rapid apoptosis could exist at the level of the endothelial cells, that they might commit suicide and thereby affect vascular function," says Rajagopalan.

Cell suicide (apoptosis) and damage to the cells lining the blood vessels (the endothelial cells) were demonstrated in the CFS and fibromyalgia spinal fluid studies (page 66).

Recent additional studies in chronic fatigue syndrome have also found "direct evidence" of endothelial dysfunction in both the large and small vessels of patients with CFS, as the following study concludes (Newton, 2011). The authors state, "This evidence collectively points to increased cardiovascular risk in ME/CFS patients, which is borne out epidemiologically by their high mortality due to heart disease.

Large and Small Artery Endothelial Dysfunction in Chronic Fatigue Syndrome

Newton, D.J., G. Kennedy, K. K.F. Chan, C.C. Lang, J. J.F. Belch, F. Khan. 2011. Int j Cardiol (Letter to the Editor).

Introduction: There is accumulating evidence that myalgic encephalomyelitis/chronic fatigue syndrome (ME/CFS) is associated with cardiovascular symptoms including autonomic dysfunction, impaired blood pressure regulation and loss of beat-to-beat heart rate control.

Aim: The primary aim of the current study was to investigate large-vessel endothelial function in ME/CFS using flow-mediated dilatation (FMD), and to assess microvascular endothelial function using post-occlusive reactive hyperaemia, both of which have been shown to be related to cardiovascular risk and outcome.

Conclusions: We believe this is the first time that vascular endothelial dysfunction has been measured directly in ME/CFS patients, and these findings build on previous work reporting indirect markers of endothelial dysfunction, such as increased oxidative stress, inflammation and arterial stiffness. This evidence collectively points to increased cardiovascular risk in ME/CFS patients, which is borne out epidemiologically by their high mortality due to heart disease.

Another condition commonly associated with autoimmune disease is interstitial cystitis. Interstitial cystitis is a chronic inflammation of the bladder that results in a feeling of pelvic discomfort, accompanied by consistently persistent and immediate urges to urinate. A recent study demonstrated that apoptotic endothelial cells also "play an important role in the pathogenesis of interstitial cystitis," the abstract for which follows (Yamada, 2007):

Increased Number of Apoptotic Endothelial Cells in Bladder of Interstitial Cystitis Patients

Yamada, T., M. Nishimura, H. Mita. 2007. World J Urol 25(4):407-13.

Abstract: In this study, we aimed to investigate possible abnormality of bladder endothelial cells in interstitial cystitis patients by detecting morphological changes such as apoptosis in bladder endothelial cells. A bladder biopsy specimen was collected from interstitial cystitis patients immediately after hydrodistension therapy. The patients were classified into two groups on the basis of their predominant symptom, one group of patients with bladder pain and another group of patients with urinary urgency. Dissociated cells from the biopsy specimen were analyzed by flow cytometry after staining with Annexin V and an anti-CD105 antibody. Terminal deoxynucleotidyl transferase-mediated dUTP nick-end labeling (TUNEL) and electron microscopy were performed to confirm morphologic changes indicative of apoptosis. The percentage of Annexin V binding, an early apoptosis marker, was significantly higher in bladder endothelial cells from interstitial cystitis patients with pain [median 24.7% (range 15.1-77.2), n = 20, P < 0.01) than that from interstitial cystitis patients with urinary urgency [9.3% (range 0.7-19.11) n = 17) or control patients [1.5% (range 0.8-9.1), n = 7]. TUNEL staining showed apoptotic cells in microvascular endothelial cells but not in the endothelial cells of a venule. By electron microscopy, endothelial cells showed morphological changes indicative of apoptosis such as nuclear fragmentation. Our results indicate that increased apoptosis of bladder microvascular endothelial cells may play an important role in the pathogenesis of interstitial cystitis accompanied by bladder pain.

Multiple Sclerosis, Depression, and Homocysteine

The following study, done in Greece, found that Plasma Homocysteine (Hcy) was "significantly increased" in MS patients compared to controls. In the conclusion, it states, "Moderately disabled MS patients with elevated Hcy levels are particularly prone to develop depressive symptoms."

Increased Plasma Homocysteine Levels in Patients with Multiple Sclerosis and Depression

Triantafyllou, N., M.E. Evangelopoulos, V.K. Kimiskidis, E. Kararizou, F. Boufidou, K.N. Fountoulakis, M. Siamouli, C. Nikolaou, C. Sfagos, N. Vlaikidis, D. Vassilopoulos. 2008. *Ann Gen Psychiatry*; 7: 17.

Background: The aim of the study was to assess the plasma levels of homocysteine in patients with multiple sclerosis (MS) and to investigate whether an association with depression exists.

Methods: Plasma homocysteine (Hcy), vitamin B12 and plasma folate were measured in 65 moderately disabled patients with relapsing/remitting MS (RR-MS) and 60 healthy controls. All subjects were assessed with the Beck Depression Inventory (BDI).

Results: Hcy levels were significantly increased in MS patients compared to controls (13.5 ± 4.7 µmol/l vs 8.5 ± 3.1, p < 0.001). A significant correlation was found between Hcy levels and BDI scores (Pearson r = 0.3025, p < 0.05). Plasma Hcy was not related to Extended Disability Status Scale (EDSS) score, age, disease duration or vitamin B12 and folate.

Conclusion: Moderately disabled MS patients with elevated Hcy levels are particularly prone to develop depressive symptomatology. Further study is warranted in order to elucidate the prognostic and therapeutic implications of this novel finding.

Vitamin B12 acts as a coenzyme in the transformation of homocysteine to methionine. This reaction is essential to make S-adenosylmethionine (SAMe), which is involved in making certain neurotransmitters. These neurotransmitters are important in maintaining mood, explaining why depression is associated with B12 deficiency. That is why SAMe is often prescribed as an antidepressant.

The following abstract also found high levels of homocysteine and low levels of B12 in multiple sclerosis patients.

Serum Vitamin B12, Folate, and Homocysteine Levels and their Association with Clinical and Electrophysiological Parameters in Multiple Sclerosis

Kocer B., S. Engur, F. Ak, M. Yilmaz. 2009. *J Clin Neurosci* 16(3):399-403.

Abstract: Patients with multiple sclerosis (MS) may have low serum vitamin B12 and folate levels and high levels of homocysteine. We aimed to evaluate serum vitamin B12, folate, homocysteine, mean corpuscular volume (MCV), hemoglobin (Hb), and hematocrit (Hct) levels in patients with MS. We examined the relationship between these parameters and age, sex, disease type, age at onset, disease duration, Expanded Disability Status Score, immunoglobulin G (IgG) index, oligoclonal band presence, visual evoked potentials (VEP) and posterior tibial somatosensory evoked potentials (SEP). These parameters were evaluated in 35 patients during an acute attack and compared to data collected from 30 healthy individuals (control subjects). Serum vitamin B12, folate, homocysteine, Hb, and Hct levels and MCV were low in a proportion of patients with MS (20%, 14.3%, 20%, 6.7%, 3.3% and 10% respectively), whereas only vitamin B12 and folate levels were low in only 3.3% of the control subjects. Homocysteine levels were high in 20% of patients with MS but were within normal limits in the control group. Elevated Hct levels were significantly correlated (p<0.05) with prolonged posterior tibial SEP P1 and P2 latencies compared to the control subjects. Patients with MS who had prolonged VEP and posterior tibial SEP P1 and P2 latencies also had lower vitamin B12 levels compared to patients with normal latencies. Thus, we found a significant relationship between MS and vitamin B12 deficiency, and also demonstrated a relationship between vitamin B12 deficiency, VEP and posterior tibial SEP in MS.

Homocysteine also plays a role in the cell death of oligodendrocytes. Oligodendrocytes are cells that coat axons in the central nervous system with their cell membrane, called myelin, producing the so-called myelin sheath. The study entitled "Homocysteine and folate deficiency sensitize oligodendrocytes to the cell death-promoting effects of a presenillin-1 mutation and amyloid beta-peptide" states, "These findings demonstrate an adverse effect of homocysteine on oligodendrocytes and suggest roles for homocysteine and folate deficiency in the white matter damage in Alzheimer's disease and related neurodegenerative disorders," (Pak, 2003). Without vitamin B12, folate becomes trapped in the body in a metabolically useless form.

Heart Disease in India and Homocysteine

As we have learned, India is the diabetic capital of the world. Another surprising fact is that India also leads the world in heart disease. India is responsible for 60% of the world's heart disease. Commenting on why Indians are more at risk for heart disease, Dr. Shashank Shah, author of a new research report presented at a World Congress event for Obesity and Metabolic Diseases in Los Angeles, stated, "We found that Indians are grossly deficient in vitamin B12, which is a crucial cardio-protective factor in the body. Vitamin B12 is usually found in food that comes from animals, like fish, meat, poultry, milk and milk products. However, since a lot of Indians are vegetarians, they do not get adequate amounts of vitamin B12 in their diet. When vitamin B12 levels fall, homocysteine levels increase. The latter is known to cause atherosclerosis (hardening and narrowing of the arteries), as well as an increased risk of heart attacks, strokes and blood clot formation," noted Dr. Shah in his report (Suryanarayan, 2010).

Dr. Shah is not alone in his findings. The following excerpt came from *The Times* of India: "Widespread deficiency of vitamin B12 among vegetarians is leading to a growing incidence of stroke and heart attacks among young people, warn doctors. Deficiency of Vitamin B12 increases the concentration of a chemical called homocysteine in the blood, which causes blocks in arteries and veins. These blocks, in turn, are responsible for heart attacks and strokes. 'More and more young people are having heart attacks and falling prey to strokes. Invariably, it is a vitamin B12 deficiency caused by a pure vegetarian diet that is leading to this condition,' said Sudhir Kothari, neurologist at Poona Hospital," (Polanki, 2004). Rustom S. Wadia, neurologist at Ruby Hall Clinic, also agrees, saying, "There is no doubt that it is a huge phenomenon. Nearly 70 percent of vegetarians have vitamin B12 deficiency. And 70 percent of the cases of strokes that I have come across are due to this deficiency."

The following abstract shows how prevalent low B12 and high homocysteine is in India. Even with an extremely low limit tested for B12 (150 pg/mL), it was found that *81%* of the urban middle class group had low B12, and *79%* had hyperhomocysteinemia.

Vitamin B12 Deficiency and Hyperhomocysteinemia in Rural and Urban Indians

Yajnik, C.S., S.S. Deshpande, H.G. Lubree, S.S. Naik, D.S. Bhat, B.S. Uradey, J.A. Deshpande, S.S. Rege, H. Refsum, J.S. Yudkin. 2006. *JAPI* 54:775-82.

Background: Low vitamin B12 concentration in South Asian Indians is common, but the exact prevalence is not known.

Aim: To investigate prevalence and associations of low vitamin B12 concentration and hyperhomocysteinemia in rural and urban Indian men living in and around Pune, Maharashtra.

Method: We studied 441 middle-aged men (149 rural, 142 slum and 150 urban middle-class residents, mean age 39 y). Data on lifestyle, socio-economic status, nutrition and medical history were obtained. Circulating concentrations of vitamin B12, folate, ferritin, total homocysteine (tHcy), and haematological indices, and cardiovascular risk variables were measured.

Results: Median plasma B12 concentration was low (110 pmol/L): Overall, 67% of men had low vitamin B12 concentration (<150 pmol/L) and 58% had hyperhomocysteinemia (>15 μmol/L). Of the urban middle class, 81% had low vitamin B12 concentration and 79% had hyperhomocysteinemia. Low vitamin B12 concentration contributed 28% to the risk of hyperhomocysteinemia (population attributable risk) while low red cell folate contributed 2%. Vegetarians had 4.4 times (95%CI 2.1, 9.4) higher risk of low vitamin B12 concentrations and 3.0 times (95%CI 1.4, 6.5) higher risk of hyperhomocysteinemia compared to those who ate non-vegetarian foods frequently. Urban middle-class residence was an additional independent risk factor of hyperhomocysteinemia (odds ratio 7.6 (95%CI 2.5, 22.6), compared to rural men). Low vitamin B12 concentration was related to lower blood haemoglobin concentration and higher mean corpuscular volume, but macrocytic anemia was rare.

Conclusion: Low vitamin B12 concentration and hyperhomocysteinemia are common in Indian men, particularly in vegetarians and urban middle class residents. Further studies are needed to confirm these findings in other parts of India.

Congestive Heart Failure and Homocysteine

Elevated homocysteine has also been linked to congestive heart failure (CHF), as is demonstrated by the following study which concludes that "increased plasma homocysteine level independently predicts risk of development of CHF…" Chronic fatigue syndrome patients have been shown to die from heart failure at a significantly lower age, i.e. 58.7 years, versus those in the general U.S. population, i.e. 83.1 years (Jason, 2006).

Plasma Homocysteine and Risk for Congestive Heart Failure in Adults Without Prior Myocardial Infarction

Vasan, R.S., A. Beiser, R.B. D'Agostino, D. Levy, J. Selhub, P.F. Jaques, I.H. Rosenberg, P.W.F. Wilson. 2003. J Amer Med Assoc 289(10):1251-7.

Context: Elevated plasma homocysteine levels are associated with increased risk of vascular disease. It is unclear whether elevated homocysteine levels are a risk factor for congestive heart failure (CHF).

Objective: To study prospectively the association between nonfasting plasma homocysteine and incidence of CHF.

Conclusions: An increased plasma homocysteine level independently predicts risk of the development of CHF in adults without prior myocardial infarction. Additional investigations are warranted to confirm these findings.

Estrogen and Homocysteine

Prior to menopause women have a reduced risk of heart disease compared with men the same age. After menopause, due to declining levels of estrogen, the risk of heart disease in women rises yearly until it is equal to that of a male.

Studies show that the protective effects of estrogen are due to its ability to lower homocysteine.

These study findings were officially recognized with a recently published statement of the Third National Health and Examination Survey (NHANES), "Higher estrogen status is associated with a decreased mean serum total homocysteine concentration-independent of nutritional status or muscle mass. It's a dramatic demonstration of the relationship between estrogen and homocysteine concentrations," stated a NHANES researcher (U.S. Department of Agriculture, 2002).

Connective Tissue and Homocysteine

"Connective tissue is a glue-like material or matrix that connects the cells that make up the body's tissues. Connective tissue gives the body's tissues and organs strength, form, and flexibility. Connective tissue also provides nutrients to tissue and aids in the special functions of certain tissues. For instance, connective tissue in joints gives them the ability to move. Connective tissue is composed of dozens of proteins and compounds containing various combinations of protein and glucose. Connective tissues' component proteins include collagens, elastins, proteoglycans, and glycoproteins. Connective tissue is found in many different organs, including the skin, bones, joints, heart, blood vessels, lungs, eyes, and ears," (Moore, 2007).

Some of the autoimmune diseases classified as connective tissue diseases are lupus, Sjögren's syndrome, Raynaud's, mixed connective tissue disease, rheumatoid arthritis, and scleroderma.

Homocysteine degrades and inhibits the formation of the three main structural components of the artery: collagen, elastin, and the proteoglycans. Homocysteine permanently degrades cysteine disulfide bridges and lysine amino acid residues in proteins, gradually affecting function and structure. Simply put, homocysteine is corrosive to long-living proteins, i.e., collagen or elastin and fibrillin. Collagen, elastin, and fibrillin are all necessary components of healthy connective tissue.

Collagen is a major component of heart valves. A disruption of collagen formation could also affect the heart valves and lead to a condition known as mitral valve prolapse (MVP). MVP is a condition where the mitral valve bulges excessively during the heartbeat. Symptoms may include fatigue, chest pain, heart palpitations, and irregular heartbeat.

MVP occurs commonly in autoimmune disease. The following study found that 75% of fibromyalgia patients had MVP.

Prevalence of Mitral Valve Prolapse in Primary Fibromyalgia: A Pilot Investigation

Pellegrino, M.J., D. Van Fossen, C. Gordon, J.M. Ryan, G.W. Waylonis. 1989. Arch Phys Med Rehabil 70(7):541-3.

Abstract: Fifty patients with primary fibromyalgia and a negative cardiovascular symptom history underwent echocardiography to determine the prevalence of mitral valve prolapse (MVP). The mean age of the population was 40 +/- 13 years (14 men, 36 women). Mitral valve prolapse was detected in 75%; 33% with myxomatous mitral valve leaflets. The prevalence of MVP in this population is significantly higher (p less than 0.0001) than in the general population. Primary fibromyalgia and MVP may be part of a more generalized connective tissue abnormality characterized by distinct genetically determined variants.

In addition to MVP, collagen disruption could affect the temporomandibular joints and lead to temporomandibular joint disorder (TMJ). The jaw joints are also made of collagen, and TMJ results when the temporomandibular joints are prevented from functioning properly. This inability to function can result in pain ranging from a dull ache in front of the ears to debilitating jaw pain and dysfunction. As with MVP, TMJ is also common in autoimmune disease.

MVP is associated with another condition common in autoimmune disease; hypermobile joints. In the study entitled "Mitral valve prolapse and joint hypermobility: evidence for a systemic connective tissue abnormality" it was stated that, "The results support previous evidence of an association between mitral valve prolapse and benign hypermobility of the joints," (Pitcher, 1982).

Joint hypermobility, in turn, is associated with pelvic organ prolapse. Pelvic organ prolapse occurs when one or more of the pelvic organs (bladder, uterus, vagina, or rectum) descend and protrude out through the opening of the vagina. The study entitled "Pelvic organ prolapse and collagen-associated disorders" stated that, "Pelvic organ prolapse (POP) and other disorders, such as varicose veins and joint hypermobility, have been associated with changes in collagen strength and metabolism," (Lammers, 2012). The study concluded that, "POP and other collagen-associated disorders may have a common aetiology, originating at the molecular level of the collagens."

The study "A Collagen Defect in Homocystinuria" states, "It is concluded that homocysteine interferes with the formation of intermolecular cross-links that help stabilize the collagen macromolecular network ..." (Kang, 1973). This would explain the loss of collagen strength originating at the molecular level in the previous study's findings.

Pregnancy and Homocysteine

The following study from Norway demonstrated that the risk of prematurely giving birth was 38% higher in women with high plasma homocysteine levels compared to women with low levels (Vollset, 2000). The study, which included nearly 6,000 women, also found that there was a significant correlation between several other complications of pregnancy and elevated homocysteine levels, including: stillbirth, preeclampsia, newborns with very low birth weights, neural tube defects, and clubfoot.

Plasma Total Homocysteine, Pregnancy Complications, and Adverse Pregnancy Outcomes: the Hordaland Homocysteine Study
Vollset, S.E., H. Refsum, L.M. Irgens, B.M. Emblem, A. Tverdal, H.K. Gjessing, A.L.B. Monsen, P.M. Ueland. 2000. *Am J Clin Nutr* 70(4):962-8.

Background: Total homocysteine (tHcy) measured in serum or plasma is a marker of folate status and a risk factor for cardiovascular disease.

Objective: Our objective was to investigate associations between tHcy and complications and adverse outcomes of pregnancy.

Design: Plasma tHcy values measured in 1992–1993 in 5883 women aged 40–42 y were compared with outcomes and complications of 14492 pregnancies in the same women that were reported to the Medical Birth Registry of Norway from 1967 to 1996.

Results: When we compared the upper with the lower quartile of plasma tHcy, the adjusted risk for preeclampsia was 32% higher [odds ratio (OR): 1.32; 95% CI: 0.98, 1.77; P for trend = 0.02], that for prematurity was 38% higher (OR: 1.38; 95% CI: 1.09, 1.75; P for trend = 0.005), and that for very low birth weight was 101% higher (OR: 2.01; 95% CI: 1.23, 3.27; P for trend = 0.003). These associations were stronger during the years closest to the tHcy determination (1980–1996), when there was also a significant relation between tHcy concentration and stillbirth (OR: 2.03; 95% CI: 0.98, 4.21; P for trend = 0.02). Neural tube defects and clubfoot had significant associations with plasma tHcy. Placental abruption had no relation with tHcy quartile, but the adjusted OR when tHcy concentrations >15 µmol/L were compared with lower values was 3.13 (95% CI: 1.63, 6.03; P = 0.001).

Conclusion: Elevated tHcy concentration is associated with common pregnancy complications and adverse pregnancy outcomes.

To reiterate, the study concluded that, "Elevated homocysteine concentration is associated with common pregnancy complications and adverse pregnancy outcomes."

Nitric Oxide and Homocysteine

Nitric oxide is an important "messenger molecule" in the body. It can be either beneficial or toxic, depending on the body's ability to properly regulate it. In our blood vessels, nitric oxide can "signal" the surrounding arterial tissues and cause them to relax. This will lower blood pressure and expand narrow blood vessels leading to improved circulation. Increased blood flow will bring more oxygen to our cells and tissues and this will, in turn, lead to more energy and even better brain function.

The beneficial properties of nitric oxide are diverse. It is a key ingredient in many erectile dysfunction products because it stimulates penile blood flow. It helps the immune system fight off infection and cancer cells, and in the brain it helps cells communicate properly.

An excess of nitric oxide, though, will react with O2-, a potent free radical, and form peroxynitrite, a powerful oxidant. Peroxynitrite is known to damage cells through multiple mechanisms.

Vitamin B12 neutralizes excess nitric oxide and prevents it from combining with O2- and forming peroxynitrite. The following studies are evidence that, due to a lack of B12, nitric oxide is playing a detrimental role in autoimmune disease.

1. Nagy, G., A. Koncz, T. Telarico, D. Fernandez, B. Ersek, E. Buzás, A. Perl. 2010. Central role of nitric oxide in the pathogenesis of rheumatoid arthritis and systemic lupus erythematosus. *Arthritis Res Ther* 12(3):210.

2. Giovannoni, G., N.C. Silver, J. O'Riordan, R.F. Miller, S.J. Heales, J.M. Land, M. Elliot, M. Feldmann, D.H. Miller, E.J. Thompson. 1999. Increased urinary nitric oxide metabolites in patients with

multiple sclerosis correlates with early and relapsing disease. *Mult Scler* 5(5):335-41.

3. Wanchu, A., M. Khullar, A. Sud, P. Bambery. 2000. Elevated nitric oxide production in patients with Sjögren's syndrome. *Clin Rheumatol* 19(5):360-4.

4. Pall, M.L. 2002. Levels of the nitric oxide synthase product citrulline are elevated in sera of chronic fatigue syndrome patients. *J Chro Fatigue Synd* 10(3/4):37-41.

5. Koskela, L.R., N.P. Wiklund. 2007. Nitric Oxide in the Painful Bladder/Interstitial Cystitis. *J Urol Urogynäkol* 14(1):18-9.

6. Broderick, K.E., V. Singh, S. Zhuang, A. Kambo, J.C. Chen, V.S. Sharma, R.B. Pilz, G.R. Boss. 2005. Nitric Oxide Scavenging by the Cobalamin (B12) Precursor Cobinamide. *J Biol Chem* 280(10):8678-85.

Nitric Oxide may also play a role in the intolerance to heat that many autoimmune patients suffer with. In a study published in Neurology, researchers from the Netherlands and Russia monitored 10 people with multiple sclerosis that had heat induced fatigue (Beenakker, 2001). The patients were cooled with special clothing and a sharp decrease in levels of fatigue was reported. But, the researchers noted, inner body temperatures did not drop during the experiment. This was to be expected they said, considering the body's mechanisms for keeping core temperatures stable.

Instead, they pointed to nitric oxide levels, which dropped in the patients who had been cooled. The following study showed that nitric oxide does indeed play a role in the control of body temperature.

Nitric Oxide and Body Temperature Control

Gerstberger, R. 1999. News Physiol Sci 14(1):30-6.

Abstract: Pharmacological studies of thermoregulatory effector and neuronal responses indicate that nitric oxide (NO) may have differential roles in the control of body temperature and during fever. Histochemical analysis of site-specific changes in NO synthase activity in defined states of thermal stimulation appears a promising approach to unravel the underlying hypothalamic neuronal cytoarchitecture.

Homocysteine can also cause nitric oxide to become dysfunctional and generate superoxide. The study entitled "Dysfunction of Endothelial Nitric Oxide Synthase and Atherosclerosis" explains how this process begins (Kawashima, 2004). It states that, "Under conditions in which vascular tissue levels of tetrahydrobiopterin, a cofactor for nitric oxide synthase are deficient or lacking, endothelial nitric oxide synthase becomes dysfunctional and produces superoxide rather than nitric oxide." So, a lack of tetrahydrobiopterin would lead to dysfunctional nitric oxide. The paper "Homocysteine impairs coronary artery endothelial function by inhibiting tetrahydrobiopterin in patients with hyperhomocysteinemia" demonstrated that, "Plasma level of nitric oxide and tetrahydrobiopterin were significantly lower in patients with hyperhomocysteinemia than in controls," (He, 2011).

Nitric oxide (NO) has also been implicated in another condition associated with autoimmune disease, endometriosis. Endometriosis is defined as the growth of endometrial tissue outside the uterine cavity. This excess growth pattern can lead to diverse symptoms, such as pelvic pain, infertility, and heavy bleeding. According to a study conducted by researchers at the National Institute of Child Health and Human Development, the George Washington University, and the Endometriosis Association, women with endometriosis were over a hundred times more likely to have chronic fatigue syndrome than the general population of U.S. women (NIH, 2002). Hypothyroidism was seven times more common and fibromyalgia was twice as likely in the women with endometriosis. The researchers also found an increased risk for lupus, Sjögren's, rheumatoid arthritis, and multiple sclerosis among the women with endometriosis.

Nitric oxide regulates vascular endothelial growth factor (VEGF). VEGF is a signal protein produced by cells that stimulates angiogenesis. Angiogenesis is the formation of new blood vessels. Without proper instruction from VEGF, endothelial cells can be stimulated to proliferate and migrate. New blood vessel formation has long been a recognized feature of endometriosis, often clearly visible by laparoscopy.

In the research paper "Nitric oxide and angiogenesis" it is stated that, "Elevation of NOS (nitric oxide synthase) activity in correlation with angiogenesis and tumor progression has been extensively reported in experimental and human tumors," (Cooke, 2002). The following study found that nitric oxide was increased in the endometrial tissues of women with endometriosis.

Nitric Oxide Synthesis is Increased in the Endometrial Tissue of Women With Endometriosis

Wu, M.Y., K.H. Chao, J.H. Yang, T.H. Lee, Y.S. Yang, H.N. Ho. 2003. *Hum Reprod* 18(12):2688-74.

Background: Previous studies have shown that peritoneal macrophages from women with endometriosis produce excess nitric oxide (NO). This study was designed to quantify the amount of NO and determine the expression of endothelial (eNOS) and inducible NO synthases (iNOS) in women with and without endometriosis.

Methods: An enzyme linked immunosorbent assay (ELISA) was performed on endometrial tissues obtained from controls (myoma, n = 30) and on eutopic/ectopic endometrial tissues from endometriosis patients (n = 34) to evaluate eNOS and iNOS protein concentrations in these endometrial tissues. A rapid response chemiluminescence analyser was used to measure NO directly in fresh endometrial tissues.

Results: Mean (± SEM) levels of NO were significantly increased in the endometrial tissues of women with endometriosis (13.2 ± 7.8 versus 19.8 ± 12.6 nmol/g tissue; P = 0.016). Apparently higher levels of NO were found in ectopic compared with eutopic endometrium (P = 0.057). Endometrial tissues of women with endometriosis appeared to contain more iNOS than those of controls (3.6 ± 2.2 versus 8.6 ± 12.2 pg/μg protein; P = 0.06), but no significant difference was found in eNOS levels.

Conclusions: Greater amounts of NO and NOS are present in the endometrial tissues of women with endometriosis, implying a possible role for NO in the pathogenesis of endometriosis.

This next study concluded that, "An increased peritoneal level of nitric oxide is a common alteration in endometriosis, endometriosis-associated infertility and idiopathic infertility and may be associated with the pathogenesis of these diseases," (Dong, 2001). Peritoneal fluid is a liquid that is made in the abdominal cavity to lubricate the tissue that lines the abdominal wall and pelvic cavity.

Increased Nitric Oxide in Peritoneal Fluid from Women with Idiopathic Infertility and Endometriosis

Dong, M., Y. Shi, Q. Cheng, M. Hao. 2001. J Repro Med 46(10):887-91.

Objective: To verify whether nitric oxide in peritoneal fluid is associated with endometriosis and infertility.

Study Design: Twenty-five women with idiopathic infertility and 38 with endometriosis were recruited, and 18 cases of uterine myomata and 2 cases of ovarian cyst served as controls. Peritoneal fluid samples were aspirated from the pouch of Douglas during laparoscopy or laparotomy. Metabolites of nitric oxide (nitrite and nitrate) in peritoneal fluid were determined by a method using nitrate reductase and the Griess reaction.

Results: Peritoneal concentrations of nitrate/nitrite in both infertile women (42.02 +/- 12.98 mmol/L) and patients with endometriosis (41.75 +/- 16.42 mmol/L) were significantly higher than that in controls (33.96 +/- 13.07, $P < .05$ for both). No significant difference in peritoneal nitrate/nitrite level was found between infertile women and patients with endometriosis ($P > .5$). Peritoneal levels of nitrate/nitrite were comparable among patients with endometriosis at different stages ($P > .5$). Patients with endometriosis had more peritoneal fluid than controls and idiopathic infertile women, while controls and idiopathic infertile women had comparable amounts of peritoneal fluid.

Conclusion: An increased peritoneal level of nitric oxide is a common alteration in endometriosis, endometriosis-associated infertility and idiopathic infertility and may be associated with the pathogenesis of these diseases.

The following study found that VEGF was also "significantly higher in endometriotic lesions."

Higher Expression of Vascular Endothelial Growth Factor (VEGF) and its Receptor VEGFR-2 (Flk-1) and Metalloproteinase-9 (MMP-9) in a Rat Model of Peritoneal Endometriosis is Similar to Cancer Diseases

Machado, D.E., P.T. Berardo, C.Y. Palmero, L.E. Nasciutti. 2010. J Exp Clin Canc Res 29:4.

Background: Endometriosis is a common disease characterized by the presence of a functional endometrium outside the uterine cavity, causing pelvic pain, dysmenorrheal, and infertility. This disease has been associated to development of different types of malignancies; therefore new blood vessels are essential for the survival of the endometrial implant. Our previous observations on humans showed that angiogenesis is predominantly found in rectosigmoid endometriosis, a deeply infiltrating disease. In this study, we have established the experimental model of rat peritoneal endometriosis to evaluate the process of angiogenesis and to compare with eutopic endometrium.

Methods: We have investigated the morphological characteristics of these lesions and the vascular density, VEGF and its receptor Flk-1 and MMP-9 expression, and activated macrophage distribution, using immunohistochemistry and RT-PCR.

Results: As expected, the auto-transplantation of endometrium pieces into the peritoneal cavity is a well-established method for endometriosis induction in rats. The lesions were cystic and vascularized, and demonstrated histological hallmarks of human pathology, such as endometrial glands and stroma. The vascular density and the presence of VEGF and Flk-1 and MMP-9 were significantly higher in endometriotic lesions than in eutopic endometrium, and confirmed the angiogenic potential of these lesions. We also observed an increase in the number of activated macrophages (ED-1 positive cells) in the endometriotic lesions, showing a positive correlation with VEGF.

Conclusion: The present endometriosis model would be useful for investigation of the mechanisms of angiogenesis process involved in the peritoneal attachment of endometrial cells, as well as of the effects of therapeutic drugs, particularly with antiangiogenic activity.

This final study concluded that, "NO modulates VEGF-induced angiogenesis and vascular permeability in vivo."

Predominant Role of Endothelial Nitric Oxide Synthase in Vascular Endothelial Growth Factor-Induced Angiogenesis and Vascular Permeability

Fukumura, D., T. Gohongi, A. Kadambi, Y. Izumi, J. Ang, C.O. Yun, D.G. Buerk, P.L. Huang, R.K. Jain. 2001. P Natl Acad Sci USA 98(5):2604-9.

Abstract: Nitric oxide (NO) plays a critical role in vascular endothelial growth factor (VEGF)-induced angiogenesis and vascular hyperpermeability. However, the relative contribution of different NO synthase (NOS) isoforms to these processes is not known. Here, we evaluated the relative contributions of endothelial and inducible NOS (eNOS and iNOS, respectively) to angiogenesis and permeability of VEGF-induced angiogenic vessels. The contribution of eNOS was assessed by using an eNOS-deficient mouse, and iNOS contribution was assessed by using a selective inhibitor [l-N6-(1-iminoethyl) lysine, l-NIL] and an iNOS-deficient mouse. Angiogenesis was induced by VEGF in type I collagen gels placed in the mouse cranial window. Angiogenesis, vessel diameter, blood flow rate, and vascular permeability were proportional to NO levels measured with microelectrodes: Wild-type (WT) ≥ WT with l-NIL or iNOS−/− > eNOS−/− ≥ eNOS−/− with l-NIL. The role of NOS in VEGF-induced acute vascular permeability increase in quiescent vessels also was determined by using eNOS- and iNOS-deficient mice. VEGF superfusion significantly increased permeability in both WT and iNOS−/− mice but not in eNOS−/− mice. These findings suggest that eNOS plays a predominant role in VEGF-induced angiogenesis and vascular permeability. Thus, selective modulation of eNOS activity is a promising strategy for altering angiogenesis and vascular permeability in vivo.

Vascular endothelial growth factor (VEGF) is a potent angiogenic and vascular permeabilizing factor. VEGF plays a critical role in both physiological and pathological angiogenesis. Nitric oxide (NO) is known to mediate many physiological and pathological functions, including angiogenesis and vascular permeability. There are three isoforms of NO synthase (NOS): neuronal NOS (nNOS, also referred to as type I NOS), inducible NOS (iNOS, type II NOS), and endothelial NOS (eNOS, type III NOS). These three isoforms of NOS are distributed and regulated differently. VEGF promotes NO production and also induces eNOS and iNOS expression in vascular endothelial cells in vitro. Furthermore, inhibition of in vivo NO production results in reduced angiogenesis and vascular permeability induced by VEGF. However, the relative contribution of the individual isoforms of NOS and the absolute amount of NO involved in these different functions in vivo are not known. Thus, in this study, we evaluated the relative contributions of eNOS and iNOS in VEGF-induced angiogenesis and vascular permeability using a collagen gel quantitative angiogenesis assay and eNOS- and iNOS-deficient mice as well as the iNOS selective inhibitor l-N6-(1-iminoethyl) lysine (I-NIL).

At this point, a logical conclusion to come to would be the possibility that there may be a correlation to the angiogenesis found in endometriosis, due to the improper regulation of vascular endothelial growth factor by nitric oxide, and cancer. In fact, women with endometriosis are at a higher risk of developing certain cancers, such as breast cancer. Are nitric oxide and vascular endothelial growth factor linked to breast cancer also? Studies show that this is indeed the case. The following study found that nitric oxide and vascular endothelial growth factor are involved in breast cancer and that this involvement correlates with "metastasis and poor prognosis," (Nakamura, 2006a).

Nitric Oxide in Breast Cancer: Induction of Vascular Endothelial Growth Factor-C and Correlation with Metastasis and Poor Prognosis

Nakamura, Y., H. Yasuoka, M. Tsuijmoto, K. Yoshidome, M. Nakamura, K. Kakudo. 2006a. *Clin Cancer Res* 12(4):1201-7.

Purpose: Metastasis to regional lymph nodes through the lymphatic vessels is a common step in the progression of cancer. Recent evidence suggests that tumor production of vascular endothelial growth factor-C (VEGF-C) promotes lymphagiogenesis, which in turn promotes lymphatic metastasis. Nitric oxide (NO) may also increase metastatic ability in human cancers.

Experimental Design: Nitrite/nitrate levels and VEGF C production were assessed in MDA-MB-231 breast cancer cells after induction and/or inhibition of NO synthesis. Formation of nitrotyrosine, a biomarker for peroxynitrate formation from NO in vivo, was analyzed in primary human breast carcinoma with long-term follow-up. The relationship between nitrotyrosine levels and lymph node status, VEGF-C immunoreactivity, and other established clinicopathologic variables, as well as prognosis, was analyzed.

Results: Production of nitrite/nitrate and VEGF-C in MDA-MB-231 cells was increased by treatment with the NO donor DETA NONOate. The NO synthase inhibitor N(G)-nitro-l-arginine methyl ester eliminated this increase. High-grade nitrotyrosine staining was observed in 57.5% (65 of 113) of the invasive breast carcinomas. Nitrotyrosine levels were significantly correlated with VEGF-C immunoreactivity and lymph node metastasis. Survival curves determined by the Kaplan-Meier method showed that high nitrotyrosine levels were associated with reduced disease-free and overall survival. In multivariate analysis, high nitrotyrosine levels emerged as a significant independent predictor for overall survival.

Conclusions: Our data showed a role for NO in stimulating VEGF-C expression in vitro. Formation of its biomarker nitrotyrosine was also correlated with VEGF-C expression and lymph node metastasis. Furthermore, high nitrotyrosine levels may serve as a significant prognostic factor for long-term survival in breast cancer.

In addition to endometriosis, autoimmune sufferers are also at an increased risk of developing certain types of cancer, such as breast and endometrial cancer. They also have an increased risk of lymphoma, a cancer that originates from white blood cells called lymphocytes and spreads from one lymph node to another. For example, according to the Johns Hopkins Lupus Center, lupus patients have a greater risk of developing breast, lung, cervical, and endometrial cancer and Sjögren's and lupus patients are both at a greater risk of developing lymphoma, (Johns Hopkins Lupus Center, 2012).

Vascular endothelial growth factor and nitric oxide were also found in the next study to correlate with lymph node metastasis in papillary thyroid carcinoma (PTC) (Nakamura, 2006b). The researchers concluded that, "NO may induce lymph node metastasis via VEGF-D stimulation in PTC."

Nitric Oxide in Papillary Thyroid Carcinoma: Induction of Vascular Endothelial Growth Factor D and Correlation with Lymph Node Metastasis

Nakamura, Y., H. Yasuoka, H. Zuo, Y. Takamura, A. Miyauchi, M. Nakamura, K. Kakudo. 2006b. J Clin Endocr Metab 91(4):1582-5.

Purpose: Vascular endothelial growth factor-D (VEGF-D) plays an important role in lymph node metastasis via lymphangiogenesis in papillary thyroid carcinoma (PTC). Although PTC metastasizes to regional lymph nodes at a high frequency, the regulation of VEGF-D expression is largely unknown.

Experimental Design: Nitrite/nitrate levels and VEGF-D production were assessed in K1 papillary thyroid carcinoma cells after induction and/or inhibition of nitric oxide (NO) synthesis. Formation of nitrotyrosine, a biomarker for peroxynitrate formation from NO in vivo, was analyzed in primary human PTC.

Results: The production of nitrite/nitrate and VEGF-D in K1 cells was increased by treatment with the NO donor, (Z)-1-[N-(2-aminoethyl)-N-(2-ammonioethyl)amino]diazen-1-ium-1,2-diolate (DETA NONOate). The NO synthase inhibitor NG-nitro-l-arginine methyl ester inhibited the increase in nitrate/nitrite and eliminated the increase in VEGF-D. High-grade nitrotyrosine staining was observed in 51.8% (29 of 56) of PTCs. Nitrotyrosine levels were significantly correlated with VEGF-D immunoreactivity and lymph node metastasis.

Conclusions: Our data showed a role for NO in stimulating VEGF-D expression in vitro. The formation of its biomarker, nitrotyrosine, was also correlated with VEGF-D expression in human PTC. NO may induce lymph node metastasis via VEGF-D stimulation in PTC.

As far as the autoimmune disease process is concerned, we shouldn't lose sight of the fact that cancerous cell growth begins with the inflammation created by homocysteine in endothelial cells. By interfering with a necessary cofactor for nitric oxide, tetrahydrobiopterin, endothelial nitric oxide synthase becomes dysfunctional and produces superoxide rather than nitric oxide. This results in the inability to properly regulate vascular endothelial growth factor. In relation to this, we would expect to see elevated homocysteine levels in metastatic breast cancer. The following study on homocysteine and metastatic breast cancer states, "Women with metastatic disease had significantly higher homocysteine concentrations compared to controls..." (Makris, 2001).

Raised Plasma Homocysteine Levels in Women with Metastatic Breast Cancer

Makris, A., H. Cladd, R.J. Burcombe, J.M. Smith, M. Makris, 2001. Proc Am Soc Clin Oncol 20:Abstract 179.

Abstract: It is well recognised that patients with malignancy have an increased risk of venous thromboembolic disease. The pathophysiology of this association has not been precisely defined. Recently hyperhomocysteinemia has become established as one of the commonest conditions associated with venous and arterial thrombosis. We examined the prevalence of hyperhomocysteinemia in women with early and advanced breast cancer. Three groups of women were studied: Group 1: healthy female controls (n=21), Group 2: early breast cancer (n=30) and Group 3: metastatic breast cancer (n=39). In the women with breast cancer all samples were collected prior to chemotherapy. The homocysteine concentration was estimated in plasma using the Abbott IMx immunoassay method. All samples were separated within 1 hour of collection. The mean (SD) plasma homocysteine levels were Group 1 - 7.9[Micro]mol/l (1.9), Group 2 - 9.57[Micro]mol/l (5.6) and Group 3 - 11.4[Micro]mol/l (5.2). 35.9% of patients with metastatic and 13.3% with early breast cancer had plasma homocysteine concentrations above the upper limit of normal. Women with metastatic disease had significantly higher plasma homocysteine concentrations compared to controls (p<0.005) or women with early breast cancer (p<0.05). No difference was observed when women with early breast cancer were compared to controls (p=0.32). We conclude that hyperhomocysteinaemia is common in women with metastatic breast cancer but was not observed in women with early disease where homocysteine concentrations were similar to controls. This observation could explain the high rate of venous thrombosis in women with metastatic breast cancer. Since hyperhomocysteinaemia is easily corrected with oral folic acid, a therapeutic trial of this drug as a thromboprophylactic agent is warranted.

The next study also found, "Elevated plasma Hcy (homocysteine) levels were significantly linked to increased risk of breast cancer…" (Chou, 2007). In addition, the researchers state that, "The current study results seem to suggest a possibility that the plasma Hcy levels could be a metabolic risk factor for breast cancer."

Plasma Homocysteine as a Metabolic Risk Factor for Breast Cancer: Findings from a Case-Control Study in Taiwan

Chou, Y.C., M.S. Lee, M.H. Wu, H.L. Shih, T. Yang, C.P. Yu, J.C. Yu, C.A. Sun. 2007. Breast Cancer Res Tr 101(2):199-205.

Abstract: Homocysteine (Hcy) is an intermediary product in methionine metabolism and an elevation in plasma Hcy is a sensitive biomarker for an imbalance in the integrated pathways of one-carbon metabolism. More recently, there has been interest in the potential links between total Hcy, folate and cancer. In this study, the association of plasma Hcy levels with the breast cancer risk was investigated. Questionnaire information and blood samples were taken before treatment from 146 women with newly diagnosed, histologically confirmed breast cancer and 285 age-matched control women who were admitted for health examination. Plasma levels of Hcy and folate were measured by enzyme conversion immunoassay and radioassay, respectively. Dietary intake of B-group vitamins was estimated using a semi-quantitative dietary questionnaire. Logistic regression was used to calculate odds ratios (ORs) and their 95% confidence intervals (CIs). Elevated plasma Hcy levels were significantly linked to increased risk of breast cancer (adjusted OR = 2.89, 95% CI = 1.70-4.92 for the highest tertile as compared with the lowest tertile). Moreover, a similar pattern of enhanced breast cancer risk at higher plasma Hcy levels was observed in both pre-menopausal and post-menopausal women. And this consistent pattern did not differ substantially by level of dietary intake of B-group vitamins. The current study results seem to suggest a possibility that the plasma Hcy levels could be a metabolic risk factor for breast cancer. Future studies are needed to prove causality and provide insight on the mechanism of action of Hcy in breast tumorigenesis.

Elevated homocysteine levels and vitamin B12 deficiencies are common in patients with inflammatory bowel disease (Romagnuolo, 2001; Yakut, 2010). The following study from France states that, "The prevalence of hyperhomocysteinemia is high in ulcerative colitis and Crohn's disease," (Roblin, 2006). The study also discusses the presence of "Five endoscopic lesions considered as precancerous," and the fact that "all of these patients had hyperhomocysteinemia." The researchers concluded that, "There is a possible link between colorectal cancer and hyperhomocysteinemia."

[Factors Associated with Hyperhomocysteinemia in Inflammatory Bowel Disease: Prospective Study in 81 Patients]

Roblin, X., E. Germain, J.M. Phelip, V. Ducros, J. Pofelski, F. Heluwaert, P. Oltean, J.L. Faucheron, B. Bonaz. 2006. Rev Med Interne 27(2):106-10.

Background: A high prevalence (52%) of hyperhomocysteinemia is observed in Crohn disease (CD), however it is not well documented in ulcerative colitis (UC). Furthermore, in the different works studying hyperhomocysteinemia the associated factors are different.

Aim: Prospective evaluation of hyperhomocysteinemia in inflammatory bowel disease (IBD) patients, of the risk factors and the determination of a potential risk of colorectal carcinoma in case of hyperhomocysteinemia.

Patients and Methods: IBD patients followed in our department were prospectively recruited between November 2003-September 2004. To be included patients should have passed a coloscopy in the two years. Patients with kidney failure or drugs supposed, to interfere with homocystéine metabolism (folates, vitamin B12, methotrexate) were excluded from the study. The following parameters were analysed: age, sex, clinical activity indexes (CDAI for Crohn disease and CAI for ulcerative colitis), length-extent and type of the disease (CD or UC), smoking, plasma homocystein concentration, folates and vitamin B12.

Results: Eighty-one patients (60 CD, 21 UC, mean age 43.8 +/- 17.3) were included, 30 had an active disease at inclusion and 16 were smokers. The prevalence of high homocystein concentration was 55.6%. In univariate analysis a low rate of folates was the only risk factor for a high homocystein concentration (74 vs. 52.8%; P = 0.018). Smoking was almost an associated factor. In multivariate analysis, a low rate of folate was the only risk factor of hyperhomocysteinemia, OR = 3.59 [1.27-10.17]. Five endoscopic lesions considered as precancerous were described; these patients had all a hyperhomocysteinemia.

Conclusion: The prevalence of hyperhomocysteinemia is high in UC and in CD. A low folate rate is the only risk factor observed in our study. There is a possible link between colorectal cancer and hyperhomocysteinemia. A high Plasma homocystein concentration must be search in inflammatory bowel disease patients and a substitutive treatment of folates and vitamin B12 is necessary in case of hyperhomocysteinemia.

Magnesium and Homocysteine

Homocysteine also interferes with the metabolism of magnesium. In the following study conducted at the Health Science Center in Brooklyn, it was determined that homocysteine causes a depletion of intracellular free magnesium. This study suggests the need for three B vitamins: B12, B6, and folic acid.

Magnesium is needed by the human body to carry out over 300 essential biochemical reactions. According to the National Institutes of Health, "Magnesium helps maintain normal muscle function and nerve function, keeps the heart rhythm steady, supports a healthy immune system, and keeps bones strong. Magnesium also helps regulate blood sugar levels, promotes normal blood pressure, and is known to be involved in energy metabolism and protein synthesis," (National Institutes of Health, 2009b).

Because magnesium is active in so many different processes in your body, magnesium deficiency symptoms are varied and can include: insomnia, muscle spasms, muscle twitches and soreness, difficulty swallowing, heart palpitations, extreme fatigue, back aches, chest tightness and difficulty breathing, osteoporosis, and dizziness. Dizziness is commonly caused by mineral deficiencies due to electrolyte imbalances.

Extracellular Magnesium Regulates Effects of Vitamin B6, B12 and Folate on Homocysteinemia-induced Depletion of Intracellular Free Magnesium Ions in Canine Cerebral Vascular Smooth Muscle Cells: Possible Relationship to [Ca2+]i, Atherogenesis and Stroke

Li, W, T. Zheng, J. Want, B.T. Altura, B.M. Altura. 1999. *Neurosci Lett* 274(2):83-6.

Homocysteine (HC) at concentrations of from 0.05 to 1.0 mM caused dose-dependent loss of [Mg2+]i in cultured cerebral vascular smooth muscle cells (VSMC), whereas cysteine and methionine (its metabolic products) failed to interfere with changes in [Mg2+]i. HC, methionine and cysteine did not produce any changes in [Ca2+]i. Lowering [Mg2+]o to 0.3 mM resulted in elevation of [Ca2+]i and loss of [Mg2+]i. Depletion of [Mg2+]i, induced by HC, was potentiated by low Mg2+. Preincubation of these cells with vitamin B6, vitamin B12, folic acid, alone, did not alter [Ca2+]i or [Mg2+]i. Likewise, concomitant addition of vitamin B6, vitamin B12, or folic acid, together with HC (1 mM) did not change the reduction in [Mg2+]i induced by HC. However, concomitant addition of HC and the three vitamins inhibited completely the loss of [Mg2+]i. Exposure of these cells to each vitamin, alone, or combination of the three vitamins failed to interfere with reduction in [Mg2+]i induced by low [Mg2+]i, but it did suppress the rise in [Ca2+]i. Interestingly, in the presence of low [Mg2+]o, the vitamin combination did not retard depletion of [Mg2+]i. The present findings are compatible with the hypothesis that an increased serum HC concentration causes abnormal metabolism of Mg2+ in cerebral VSMC, thus priming these cells for HC-induced atherogenesis, cerebral vasospasm and stroke. Our results suggest the need for the three B-vitamins, together with normal physiological levels of Mg2+, in order to prevent [Mg2+]i depletion and occlusive cerebral vascular diseases induced by homocysteinemia.

The following study found "a statistically significant decrease" in intracellular magnesium (Mg) in patients with multiple sclerosis. Erythrocytes are red blood cells.

Magnesium Concentration in Plasma and Erythrocytes in MS
Stelmasiak, Z, J. Solski, B. Jakubowska. 1995. Acta Neurol Scan 92(1):109-11.

Abstract: There are few reports of Mg in MS and none dealing with Mg content in erythrocytes. Mg concentration was determined in serum and in erythrocytes with the help of a BIOTROL Magnesium Calmagite colorimetric method (average sensitivity: 0.194 A per mmol/l) and a Hitachi autoanalyzer in 24 MS patients (7 men and 17 women, age 29-60; 37 years on average with the duration of the disease: 3-19; 11 years on average, at clinical disability stages according to the Kurtzke scale: 1-7; 3.2 on average, in remission stage. A statistically significant decrease ($p < 0.001$) of Mg concentration in erythrocytes and no changes in plasma of MS patients were found. The results obtained suggest the presence of changes in membrane of erythrocytes which could be connected with their shorter life and with affection of their function.

Another study entitled "Magnesium concentration in brains from multiple sclerosis patients" also found MS patients had significantly lower Mg (Yasui, 1990). The study states that, "The average Mg content in the CNS tissues, as well as visceral organs except for spleen, of MS patients showed a significantly lower value than that seen in control cases."

A lack of intracellular magnesium is commonly found in patients suffering with autoimmune disease.

Osteoporosis and Homocysteine

Osteoporosis, which means "porous bone," is a disease depicted by an increased risk of fractures due to weak bones. Homocysteine has been established through numerous studies to be a "strong and independent risk factor" for osteoporosis. Homocysteine may affect osteoporosis by interfering with collagen cross-linking, resulting in a defective bone matrix. The following study was done as part of The Framingham Osteoporosis Study funded by the National Institutes of Health (McLean, 2004). The age-adjusted risk for hip fracture was four times higher for men and nearly twice as high for women in the group with 25% of the highest homocysteine readings.

Homocysteine as a Predictive Factor for Hip Fracture in Older Persons

McLean, R.R., P.F. Jacques, J. Selhub, K.L. Tucker, E.J. Samelson, K.E. Broe, M.T. Hannan, L.A. Cupples, D.P. Kiel. 2004. New Engl J Med 350(20):2042-9.

Background: The increased prevalence of osteoporosis among people with homocystinuria suggests that a high serum homocysteine concentration may weaken bone by interfering with collagen cross-linking, thereby increasing the risk of osteoporotic fracture. We examined the association between the total homocysteine concentration and the risk of hip fracture in men and women enrolled in the Framingham Study.

Methods: We studied 825 men and 1174 women, ranging in age from 59 to 91 years, from whom blood samples had been obtained between 1979 and 1982 to measure plasma total homocysteine. The participants in our study were followed from the time that the sample was obtained through June 1998 for incident hip fracture. Sex-specific, age-adjusted incidence rates of hip fracture were calculated for quartiles of total homocysteine concentrations. Cox proportional-hazards regression was used to calculate hazard ratios for quartiles of homocysteine values.

Results: The mean (+/-SD) plasma total homocysteine concentration was 13.4+/-9.1 micromol per liter in men and 12.1+/-5.3 micromol per liter in women. The median duration of follow-up was 12.3 years for men and 15.0 years for women. There were 41 hip fractures among men and 146 among women. The age-adjusted incidence rates per 1000 person-years for hip fracture, from the lowest to the highest quartile for total homocysteine, were 1.96 (95 percent confidence interval, 0.52 to 3.41), 3.24 (0.97 to 5.52), 4.43 (1.80 to 7.07), and 8.14 (4.20 to 12.08) for men and 9.42 (5.72 to 13.12), 7.01 (4.29 to 9.72), 9.58 (6.42 to 12.74), and 16.57 (11.84 to 21.30) for women. Men and women in the highest quartile had a greater risk of hip fracture than those in the lowest quartile--the risk was almost four times as high for men and 1.9 times as high for women.

Conclusions: These findings suggest that the homocysteine concentration, which is easily modifiable by means of dietary intervention, is an important risk factor for hip fracture in older persons.

The following study concluded that, "An increased homocysteine level appears to be a strong and independent risk factor for osteoporotic fractures in older men and women."

Homocysteine Levels and the Risk of Osteoporotic Fracture

van Meurs, J.B., R.A. Dhonukshe-Rutten, S.M. Pluijm, K. van der Klift, R. de Jonge, J. Lindemans, L.C. de Groot, A. Hofman, J.C. Witteman, J.P. van Leeuwen, M.M. Breteler, P. Lips, H.A. Pols, A.G. Uitterlinden. 2004. New Engl J Med 350(20):233-41.

Background: Very high plasma homocysteine levels are characteristic of homocystinuria, a rare autosomal recessive disease accompanied by the early onset of generalized osteoporosis. We therefore hypothesized that mildly elevated homocysteine levels might be related to age-related osteoporotic fractures.

Methods: We studied the association between circulating homocysteine levels and the risk of incident osteoporotic fracture in 2406 subjects, 55 years of age or older, who participated in two separate prospective, population-based studies. In the Rotterdam Study, there were two independent cohorts: 562 subjects in cohort 1, with a mean follow-up period of 8.1 years; and 553 subjects in cohort 2, with a mean follow-up period of 5.7 years. In the Longitudinal Aging Study Amsterdam, there was a single cohort of 1291 subjects, with a mean follow-up period of 2.7 years. Multivariate Cox proportional-hazards regression models were used for analysis of the risk of fracture, with adjustment for age, sex, body-mass index, and other characteristics that may be associated with the risk of fracture or with increased homocysteine levels.

Results: During 11,253 person-years of follow-up, osteoporotic fractures occurred in 191 subjects. The overall multivariable-adjusted relative risk of fracture was 1.4 (95 percent confidence interval, 1.2 to 1.6) for each increase of 1 SD in the natural-log-transformed homocysteine level. The risk was similar in all three cohorts studied, and it was also similar in men and women. A homocysteine level in the highest age-specific quartile was associated with an increase by a factor of 1.9 in the risk of fracture (95 percent confidence interval, 1.4 to 2.6). The associations between homocysteine levels and the risk of fracture appeared to be independent of bone mineral density and other potential risk factors for fracture.

Conclusions: An increased homocysteine level appears to be a strong and independent risk factor for osteoporotic fractures in older men and women.

An additional study from Morocco found that homocysteine was "significantly higher" in the osteoporotic patient group than in control patients, and that homocysteine and vitamin B12 were independent risk factors for osteoporosis.

Relation of Plasma Total Homocysteine, Folate and Vitamin B12 Levels to Bone Mineral Density in Moroccan Healthy Postmenopausal Women

Ouzzif, Z., K. Oumghar, K. Sbai, A. Mounach, M. El Derouiche, A. El Maghraoui. 2012. Rheumatol Int 32(1):123-8.

Abstract: To test whether in Moroccan healthy postmenopausal women, levels of plasma total homocysteine (tHcy), folate, and vitamin B12 are related to BMD. A total of 188 volunteer postmenopausal women were recruited from our blood taking center between April 2008 and December 2008. Each subject completed a standardized questionnaire designed to document putative risk factors of osteoporosis. Bone mineral density was determined by a Lunar Prodigy Vision DXA system, and blood samples for plasma tHcy, folate, vitamin B12, and serum parathyroid hormone (PTH) were taken. Comparison between women with osteoporosis, osteopenia and normal BMD showed that the osteoporotic women were significantly older, had lower weight and height than the women of the other groups. Plasma tHcy was significantly higher in the osteoporotic group. Levels of tHcy were inversely related to BMD at the lumbar spine, at the total hip and plasma vitamin B12 and positively related to age and creatinine. Multiple regression analysis showed that age and BMI were the main predictors of BMD at the lumbar spine, whereas the main predictors of BMD at the total hip were age, BMI, plasma tHcy, and plasma vitamin B(12). tHcy and vitamin B12 are independent risk factors for osteoporosis in Moroccan healthy postmenopausal women.

Hypothyroidism and Homocysteine

In the following study, researchers concluded that homocysteine levels are elevated in hypothyroidism and that "the association of hyperhomocysteinemia and lipid abnormalities occurring in hypothyroidism may represent a dynamic atherogenic state." Atherogenic refers to "the ability to initiate or accelerate atherogenesis—the deposition of atheromas, lipids, and calcium in the arterial lumen," (Houghton Mifflin, 2007). As the abstract states, the data obtained from these experiments demonstrated that the use of thyroid hormone failed to completely normalize homocysteine levels.

Homocysteine, Hypothyroidism, and Effect of Thyroid Hormone Replacement

Catargi, B., F. Parrot-Roulaud, C. Cochet, D. Ducassou, P. Roger, A. Tabarin. 1999. *Thyroid* 9(12):1163-6.

Abstract: Elevation of total plasma concentration of homocysteine (t-Hcy) is an important and independent risk factor for cardiovascular disease. Hypothyroidism is possibly also associated with an increased risk for coronary artery disease, which may be related to atherogenic changes in lipid profile. Because hypothyroidism decreases hepatic levels of enzymes involved in the remethylation pathway of homocysteine, we prospectively evaluated fasting and postload t-Hcy in patients before and after recovery of euthyroidism. Fasting and postload t-Hcy levels were higher in 40 patients with peripheral hypothyroidism (14 with autoimmune thyroiditis and 26 treated for thyroid cancer) in comparison with those of 26 controls (13.0 +/- 7.5 vs. 8.5 +/- 2.6 micromol/L, $p < .01$, respectively, and 49.9 +/- 37.3 vs. 29.6 +/- 8.4 micromol/L $p < .001$, respectively). On univariate analysis, fasting Hcy was positively related to thyrotropin (TSH) and inversely related to folates. Multivariate analysis confirmed TSH as the strongest predictor of t-Hcy independent of age, folate, vitamin B12, and creatinine. Thyroid hormone replacement significantly decreased fasting but not postload t-Hcy. We conclude that t-Hcy is elevated in hypothyroidism. The association of hyperhomocysteinemia and lipid abnormalities occurring in hypothyroidism may represent a dynamic atherogenic state. Thyroid hormone failed to completely normalize t-Hcy. Potential benefit of treatment with folic acid in combination with thyroid hormone replacement has to be tested given that hypothyroid patients were found to have lower levels of folate.

Vision Problems Associated With Homocysteine

People with autoimmune disease often experience vision complications. Just as blood vessels leading to and from the heart and brain can be adversely affected by homocysteine, so can other blood vessels in the body. Central retinal vein occlusion (CRVO), central retinal artery occlusion (CRAO), and nonarteritic anterior ischemic optic neuropathy (NAION), are three eye conditions associated with elevated homocysteine. All three are serious conditions that can lead to vision loss. Ischemic CRVO, which usually occurs in one eye only, leads to all sorts of complications, including neovascular glaucoma and macular degeneration.

Referring to images of a fragmented 10-layer retina exposed to high levels of homocysteine, Dr. Sylvia Smith, cell biologist at the Medical College of Georgia, states in an article from *Medical News Today*, "You don't have to be a cell biologist to see there is a problem in this retina. It's terribly disrupted. A healthy retina-tissue at the back of the eye that receives light and transforms it to a neural impulse that goes to the brain is beautifully organized, horizontally and vertically."

The following study from Turkey found that homocysteine levels were "significantly higher" in patients with macular degeneration and that B12 levels were "significantly lower."

Plasma Homocysteine, Vitamin B12 and Folate Levels in Age-Related Macular Degeneration

Kamburoglu, G., K. Gumus, S. Kadayifcilar, B. Eldem. 2006. *Graefes Arch. Clin. Exp. Ophthalmol.* 244(5):565-9.

Purpose: The purpose of this study was to investigate the association of age-related macular degeneration (AMD) with plasma homocysteine, vitamin B12, and folate levels.

Methods: Sixty patients diagnosed with AMD at our clinic between March 2004 and September 2004 were assessed in a prospective cross-sectional study. Plasma homocysteine, vitamin B12, and folate levels taken after 8 h of fasting from 30 patients with exudative AMD and 30 patients with dry AMD were compared with the results of 30 age- and sex-matched healthy participants.

Results: Patients with both exudative and dry types of AMD had significantly higher plasma homocysteine levels (mean 14.19+/-3.11 micromol/l; 13.07+/-2.90 micromol/l respectively) compared with the controls (mean 10.79+/-2.56 micromol/l; ($p=0.000$ and $p=0.008$ respectively). Homocysteine levels were higher in the exudative AMD group compared with the dry AMD group, but the difference was not statistically significant ($p=0.290$). Plasma vitamin B12 levels were found to be significantly lower in the exudative AMD group (289.14+/-113.44 pg/l) compared with the controls (436.17+/-204.12 pg/l) and dry AMD group (443.47+/-190.83 pg/l; ($p=0.000$). Plasma folate levels were comparable among groups ($p=0.106$).

Conclusion: This study suggests an association between elevated plasma homocysteine and AMD regardless of the subtype. Further controlled prospective studies are needed to investigate the possible role of homocysteine in AMD and the effect of vitamin B12 and folate supplementation in this process.

The following study concluded that "increased homocysteine and low vitamin B12 were independently associated with an increased risk of AMD..."

Elevated Serum Homocysteine, Low Serum Vitamin B12, Folate, and Age-Related Macular Degeneration: the Blue Mountains Eye Study

Rochtchina, E., J.J. Wang, V.M. Flood, P. Mitchell. 2007. *Am J Ophthalmol.* 143(2):344-6.

Purpose: To assess associations between increased serum homocysteine, low vitamin B12, low folate, and age-related macular degeneration (AMD).

Design: Population-based, cross-sectional analysis.

Methods: Serum homocysteine, vitamin B12, and folate were measured in 2,335 participants of the Blue Mountains Eye Study second survey. AMD detected from retinal photographs included atrophic or neovascular lesions.

Results: After adjusting for age, gender, and smoking in logistic regression models, homocysteine >15 micromol/l was associated with an increased likelihood of AMD in participants aged <75 years (odds ratio [OR] 3.21, 95% confidence interval [95% CI] 1.09 to 9.43). A similar association was found for vitamin B12 <125 pmol/l (OR 2.30, 95% CI 1.08 to 4.89) among all participants. In participants with homocysteine < or =15 micromol/l, low serum B12 was associated with nearly four-fold higher odds of AMD (OR 3.74, 95% CI 1.06 to 13.24). Folate was not statistically significantly associated with AMD.

Conclusions: Increased homocysteine and low vitamin B12 were independently associated with an increased risk of AMD in this study population.

Homocysteine was the reason my hands felt as if someone had set them on fire. There can be no doubt that elevated homocysteine is a primary cause of so many of the deteriorating conditions associated with autoimmune disease.

Chapter 2 THE DISCOVERY

Tumor Necrosis Factor and Its Role in Autoimmune Disease

Tumor Necrosis Factor—sounds scary, doesn't it? I had heard of it, but the day I developed a deeper understanding of its role in autoimmune disease, was the day I met Eric. Eric is a 23-year-old young man that was brought to see me by his mother. He had suffered with Crohn's disease for years and had already had two surgeries at Mayo Clinic to try and alleviate his pain and suffering. At one time, this tall young man weighed only 126 pounds due to his inability to eat without extreme pain. He arrived at my home looking very skinny, pale, and a little leery. Let's just say he would most likely not have come if his mother had not brought him. They mentioned he had been giving himself daily injections of a drug called Humira® to treat his Crohn's. He had stopped after two months because he did not feel it was helping, and he was experiencing bad side effects. Among his side effects were serious skin infections that resulted in boil-like eruptions, which he had to have cut out. His doctors also put him on a three month course of antibiotics to help combat the infections. This may have only further aggravated his Crohn's disease. Antibiotic use results not only in the destruction of harmful bacteria, but also of the beneficial bacteria that reside in our gut. In the third section of this book, we explain why the destruction of beneficial bacteria is one of the factors that contribute to the development of autoimmune disease.

The following article excerpt from *The Daily Mail*, discusses the connection between antibiotic use and the development of IBS and Crohn's.

Antibiotics Increase Risk of IBS and Crohn's Disease in Children in Later Life
Borland, S. 2011. *The Daily Mail.*

Children given antibiotics are twice as likely to develop digestive problems, research shows. Those prescribed penicillin and similar medicines are more at risk from irritable bowel syndrome (IBS) and Crohn's disease. Scientists believe the drugs may encourage harmful bacteria and other organisms to grow in the gut, which trigger the conditions. A research team looked at 580,000 children over an eight-year period and examined records of their prescriptions and medical history.

The study, published in the journal Gut, showed that children prescribed at least one course of antibiotics by the time they were four were almost twice as likely to have developed IBS. They were also three and a half times more at risk of Crohn's disease, an incurable condition which causes abdominal pain, weight loss, nausea and other unpleasant symptoms.

The researchers believe antibiotics destroy 'good' bacteria and other tiny organisms known collectively as 'microflora' which help protect the gut.

This makes the intestines less tolerant of harmful bacteria, and the person is more susceptible to IBS and similar conditions. Overall, children aged three or four who had been given antibiotics were 1.84 times more likely to be diagnosed with bowel disease than those never given the drugs. And the risk of developing the illness increased by 12 percent every time the medicines were prescribed.

When Eric and his mother left, I decided to research Humira® to see why it was supposed to help with Crohn's disease. The Humira® website states, "Many patients with Crohn's disease produce too much of a protein called tumor necrosis factor (TNF) in their body. This excess attacks the intestines and other parts of the gastrointestinal (GI) tract, and can cause them to become inflamed. This can result in the pain, diarrhea, and other symptoms of Crohn's disease. Humira® belongs to a class of biologics known as TNF blockers. TNF blockers have a specific target in the body and work by binding the excess TNF to help block the inflammation that can lead to Crohn's symptoms," (Abbott Laboratories, 2010).

What is TNF? TNF is a protein produced by white blood cells. Its job is to fight infection. It's a perfectly normal part of the immune system. So, my questions were, "Why is there an excess? What is responsible for keeping it within normal limits and degrading it when necessary?" As the following abstract shows, the degradation and inactivation of TNF is performed by *pancreatic proteases*. So, if you lack pancreatic proteases, you would be a candidate for elevated levels of TNF.

Degradation and Inactivation of Plasma Tumor Necrosis Factor-alpha by Pancreatic Proteases in Experimental Acute Pancreatitis

Alsfasser, G., B. Antoniu, S.P. Thayer, A.L. Warshaw, C. Fernández-del Castillo. 2005. Pancreatology 5(1):37-43.

Conclusion: Plasma TNFalpha does not rise in experimental acute pancreatitis, and levels are significantly lower in severe pancreatitis compared to sham-operated controls. Our study demonstrates degradation and inactivation of TNFalpha by pancreatic proteases, suggesting that it is unlikely it plays an important role in the development of distant organ failure.

Cells of the immune system produce proteins called cytokines. There are different types of cytokines-including TNF. These cytokines do amazing things to fight off infection. Much like homocysteine though, if TNF is not controlled, it is capable of doing a great deal of damage to the body. Systemically, TNF acts on the hypothalamus to generate fever and suppress appetite. We've all experienced this when fighting illness, but it can happen with rheumatoid arthritis and Crohn's as well. TNF also kicks off a process called an "acute phase response." This can show up in your blood work as elevated CRP or C–Reactive Protein. In diabetes, it can cause insulin resistance. Locally, TNF can cause heat, redness, swelling, and pain—as seen in joints affected by rheumatoid arthritis.

According to an article in *Molecular Psychiatry*, "TNF has long been implicated in the immunopathogenesis of Multiple Sclerosis (MS), which is an inflammatory and demyelinating disease of the central nervous system. *In MS the magnitude of the elevation of TNF in cerebrospinal fluid mirrors the severity of the disease*," (Finsen, 2002).

"TNF appears to play a major pro-inflammatory role in SLE also," as is stated in the research article "The role of tumor necrosis factor-alpha in systemic lupus erythematosus," (Aringer, 2008).

Another class of pancreatic enzymes, serine proteases, has also been identified as immune modulators. These modulators fine-tune the immune response and prevent unwanted inflammation from damaging tissues. The following abstract outlines the role of serine proteases in the immune response.

Neutrophil Serine Proteases Fine-Tune the Inflammatory Response
Pham, C.T.N. 2008. *Int J Biochem Cell Biol.* 40(6-7):1317-1333.

Abstract: Neutrophil serine proteases are granule-associated enzymes known mainly for their function in the intracellular killing of pathogens. Their extracellular release upon neutrophil activation is traditionally regarded as the primary reason for tissue damage at the sites of inflammation. However, studies over the past several years indicate that neutrophil serine proteases may also be key regulators of the inflammatory response. Neutrophil serine proteases specifically process and release chemokines, cytokines, and growth factors, thus modulating their biological activity. In addition, neutrophil serine proteases activate and shed specific cell surface receptors, which can ultimately prolong or terminate cytokine-induced responses. Moreover, it has been proposed that these proteases can impact cell viability through their caspase-like activity and initiate the adaptive immune response by directly activating lymphocytes. In summary, these studies point to neutrophil serine proteases as versatile mediators that fine-tune the local immune response and identify them as potential targets for therapeutic interventions.

Tumor necrosis factor also plays a role in autoimmune diseases not associated with inflammation, such as chronic fatigue syndrome (CFS). Autoimmune sufferers, including CFS patients, often have unexplained symptoms such as malaise, night sweats, sore throat, swollen glands, and low-grade fevers, for no apparent reason.

Researchers at Duke University Medical Center have tracked down the cells that trigger sore, swollen glands in the throat. Small immune organs, known as lymph nodes, are found throughout the body (including the neck) and swell to help fight bacteria and viruses during an infection. The swelling occurs as the body starts producing cells to help fight the infection.

A group of cells, called 'mast cells', start the swelling. The Duke University researchers found that mast cells release tumor necrosis factor. It journeys to the lymph nodes, where it activates infection fighting cells. This would explain the swollen glands that often accompany autoimmune disease, even without an infectious agent present.

The following abstract identifies, "Dysregulated expression of tumor necrosis factor in chronic fatigue syndrome."

Dysregulated Expression of Tumor Necrosis Factor in Chronic Fatigue Syndrome: Interrelations with Cellular Sources and Patterns of Soluble Immune Mediator Expression

Patarca, R., N.G. Kilmas, S. Lugtendorf, M. Antoni, M.A. Fletcher. 1994. *Clin Infect Dis.* 18(Suppl.1):S147-53.

Abstract: Among a group of 70 individuals who met the criteria established by the Centers for Disease Control and Prevention (Atlanta) for chronic fatigue syndrome (CFS), 12%-28% had serum levels exceeding 95% of control values for tumor necrosis factor (TNF) alpha, TNF-beta, interleukin (IL) 1 alpha, IL-2, soluble IL-2 receptor (sIL-2R), or neopterin; overall, 60% of patients had elevated levels of one or more of the nine soluble immune mediators tested. Nevertheless, only the distributions for circulating levels of TNF-alpha and TNF-beta differed significantly in the two populations. In patients with CFS--but not in controls--serum levels of TNF-alpha, IL-1 alpha, IL-4, and sIL-2R correlated significantly with one another and (in the 10 cases analyzed) with relative amounts (as compared to beta-globin or beta-actin) of the only mRNAs detectable by reverse transcriptase-coupled polymerase chain reaction in peripheral-blood mononuclear cells: TNF-beta, unspliced and spliced; IL-1 beta, lymphocyte fraction; and IL-6 (in order of appearance). These findings point to polycellular activation and may be relevant to the etiology and nosology of CFS.

The following study confirms that mast cells also play a central role in interstitial cystitis.

The Mast Cell in Interstitial Cystitis: Role in Pathophysiology and Pathogenesis

Sant, G.R., D. Kempuraj, J.E. Marchand, T.C. Theoharides. 2007. Urology 69(4 Suppl):34-40.

Abstract: Current evidence from clinical and laboratory studies confirms that mast cells play a central role in the pathogenesis and pathophysiology of interstitial cystitis (IC). In this article, we focus on the role of the mast cell in IC and examine the ways in which mast cells and other pathophysiologic mechanisms are interrelated in this disease. Identifying the patients with IC who have mast cell proliferation and activation will enable us to address this aspect of disease pathophysiology in these individuals with targeted pharmacotherapy to inhibit mast cell activation and mediator release.

The powerful destructive combination of elevated homocysteine and tumor necrosis factor would clearly explain the painful features of interstitial cystitis.

Psoriasis and Psoriatic Arthritis

"Substantial evidence suggests that TNF plays a fundamental role in the pathogenesis of psoriasis and psoriatic arthritis," according to the following review from the University of Utah School of Medicine, Department of Dermatology (Krueger, 2004). Psoriasis is a chronic autoimmune disease that appears on the skin. It occurs when the immune system sends out faulty signals that speed up the growth cycle of cells. The most common form, plaque psoriasis, is commonly seen as red and white hues on the top first layer of the epidermis (skin). Psoriasis can also cause inflammation of the joints, which is known as psoriatic arthritis.

The study also states, "Aberrant regulation of TNF is involved in the development of psoriasis and psoriatic arthritis." (We have shown that TNF is regulated by proteases). Elevated levels of TNF have also been detected in the synovial fluids of patients with psoriatic arthritis. The researchers concluded, "Tumor necrosis factor plays a major role in the pathogenesis of psoriasis and psoriatic arthritis."

Potential of Tumor Necrosis Factor Inhibitors in Psoriasis and | Psoriatic Arthritis

Krueger, G., K. Callis. 2004. *Arch Dermatol.* 140:218-225.

Objectives: To summarize the role of tumor necrosis factor (TNF) in the pathogenesis of psoriasis and psoriatic arthritis (PsA) and to present the latest data on the efficacy of TNF inhibitors in these diseases.

Study Selection: Sources that described a role for TNF in the pathogenesis of psoriasis and PsA were selected based on relevance. Clinical trials that examined the efficacy of the TNF inhibitors etanercept and infliximab in psoriasis and PsA were selected.

Data Extraction: Data were extracted if they represented safety information, the American College of Rheumatology criteria for improvement, the Health Assessment Questionnaire, or the PsA response criteria. These data were abstracted independently by the authors.

Data Synthesis: Aberrant regulation of TNF is involved in the development of psoriasis and PsA. Therefore, recent intervention strategies for psoriasis and PsA have incorporated biologic agents that specifically target TNF. Etanercept and infliximab are effective at reducing disease activity and are generally well tolerated in the treatment of psoriasis and PsA.

Conclusion: Tumor necrosis factor plays a major role in the pathogenesis of psoriasis and PsA, and TNF antagonists provide clinicians with a worthy alternative to traditional therapies, which are associated with toxic effects and poor compliance.

Tumor necrosis factor is also linked to rheumatoid cachexia. Rheumatoid cachexia is a loss of muscle mass and strength with a simultaneous increase in fat mass. It is a common condition in patients with RA. In the study entitled "Tumor necrosis factor and muscle wasting: a cellular perspective" researchers concluded that, "It appears that TNF can act directly on mature muscle to accelerate protein degradation," (Reid, 2001).

Ulcerative Colitis

Tumor necrosis factor is also involved in the pathogenesis of ulcerative colitis (UC). UC is a form of inflammatory bowel disease that causes ulcers or open sores in the colon (large intestine). In the research paper entitled "Tumor Necrosis Factor in Ulcerative Colitis and Diverticular Disease Associated Colitis" it states that, "In particular, the role of tumor necrosis factor alpha (TNF-a) in UC pathogenesis has been clarified by serological and immunohistochemical studies in humans and by experimental models," (Hassan, 2007).

If TNF can cause ulcers in our colon, then logically, it could also be responsible for ulcers in oral mucosal tissue. Recurrent aphthous ulceration (RAU) or canker sores, is a common occurrence in autoimmune disease. The paper "Salivary interleukin-6 and tumor necrosis factor-alpha in patients with recurrent aphthous ulceration" states that, "Recurrent aphthous ulceration (RAU) is a well-known oral disease which seems to be mediated principally by the immune system," (Boras, 2006). The researchers found significant differences in salivary TNF between healthy controls and patients with acute RAU. No differences in salivary interleukin-6 between the groups could be found.

The study "The pancreas and inflammatory bowel diseases" identifies the connection to IBD and the pancreas (Herrlinger, 2000). It states that, "IBD patients have a markedly elevated risk for developing acute pancreatitis as well as pancreatic insufficiency."

We now have an explanation for so many of the symptoms of autoimmune disease. Tumor necrosis factor is responsible for the inflammation of the intestines in Crohn's, the swelling and pain of the joints in RA, insulin resistance in diabetes, elevated C-Reactive Protein, and the fever and loss of appetite that all of these diseases often share. It also has a direct correlation to MS.

Additionally, I learned from the Humira® website, "Humira® can cause serious side effects, including: serious infections, nervous system problems, blood problems, heart failure or worsening of heart failure, psoriasis, immune reactions, including a lupus-like syndrome, and certain types of cancer."

It would seem to make more sense to simply fix the problem at the source, rather than risk such serious side-effects of various drugs. TNF would then get back to being a benefit to our bodies, rather than a painful disease promoter. Oh, and Eric—he started on the diet in this book the same day I met him. He paid me a visit just yesterday (on his own, without his mother) and he said, "Thanks for getting this all figured out." It has only been a few weeks since he came to see me, but he is well on his way to recovery.

CHAPTER 2 THE DISCOVERY

Signs and Symptoms of Pancreatic Enzyme Deficiency Disease

We have shown that the autoimmune diseases in this book share a common cause. Many autoimmune sufferers are often diagnosed with more than one autoimmune disease and sometimes multiple diseases. This would be expected, since all of them originate from the same source. The following information shows just how common this is.

An article in *Arthritis Today* states, "New research shows that people with diabetes are nearly twice as likely to have arthritis, indicating a diabetes-arthritis connection," (Mann, 2011). In addition, a new epidemiological study from Denmark demonstrates that people with type 1 diabetes are three times more likely to develop multiple sclerosis than people without diabetes (Nielsen, 2006). Researchers from the University of Tennessee Health Sciences Center in Memphis have identified a link between hypothyroidism and type 1 diabetes. In the study, 41% of the female diabetic patients developed hypothyroidism (Muralidhara Krishna, 2011). An Israeli study titled "Fibromyalgia in diabetes mellitus" concluded "Fibromyalgia is a common finding in patients with types 1 and 2 diabetes...," (Tishler, 2003).

Reporting in the May 2006 issue of the *Journal of Rheumatology*, researchers identified an association between rheumatoid arthritis and multiple sclerosis. They state, "Since a great proportion of our patients developed MS first and subsequently RA, the best explanation for these cases is a predisposition in MS patients to develop another autoimmune disease with common etiologic cofactors." An abstract from the *Annals of the Rheumatic Diseases* found that, "Clinical hypothyroidism was observed three times more often in female RA patients than females in the general population," (Raterman, 2008).

Arthritis Today also states, "People with other rheumatic diseases, such as rheumatoid arthritis or lupus, are at greater risk for fibromyalgia. For example, about 20 to 30 percent of people with rheumatoid arthritis also develop fibromyalgia, although no one knows why," (Arthritis Today, 2009). The Lupus Foundation of America states, "Fibromyalgia affects about 30 percent of people with lupus," (Lupus Foundation of America, 2011).

The Johns Hopkins Lupus Center states, "Autoimmune thyroid disease is common in lupus," (Johns Hopkins Lupus Center, 2011). The National Fibromyalgia Association states, "Patients with established rheumatoid arthritis, lupus, and Sjögren's syndrome often develop fibromyalgia during the course of their illness," (Bennett, 2009).

The website www.boneandspine.com states, "Myasthenia gravis is associated with various autoimmune diseases, including: thyroid diseases, diabetes, rheumatoid arthritis, lupus, and demyelinating central nervous system diseases," (Singh, 2010). The Archives of Neurology states, "Myasthenia gravis has been associated with disorders of the thyroid gland…," (Donaldson, 1983). Healthy Divas, a resource center for autoimmune disease, states, "An estimated 85% of Chronic Fatigue Syndrome sufferers also have hypothyroidism," (Whitaker, 2007).

The National Institutes of Health reports that, "About 1 out of 3 people who has lupus has Raynaud's." Also, "About 9 out of 10 people who have scleroderma have Raynaud's," (National Institutes of Health, 2011). WebMD states, "For some people, Raynaud's phenomenon is the first sign of rheumatoid arthritis," (WebMD, 2011). Mayo Clinic lists scleroderma, lupus, rheumatoid arthritis, and Sjögren's syndrome as causes of secondary Raynaud's (Mayo Clinic staff, 2009). The International Scleroderma Network reports, "About twenty percent of patients with systemic scleroderma also have secondary Sjögren's syndrome," (International Scleroderma Network, 2011).

The protein findings in the spinal tap studies have shown that fibromyalgia and chronic fatigue are nearly identical, if not identical diseases. I had someone tell me once, they had suffered with fibromyalgia for 20 years, and then had been diagnosed with multiple sclerosis. It would make sense that as the body becomes more depleted of vitamin B12, enzymes, and essential amino acids, you would see increasingly severe and varying symptoms. Every individual is unique in the amount of enzymes he has to begin with, the foods he eats, the antibiotics or medications he takes, etc. If the depletion of enzymes is not as severe, one may only develop rosacea for instance. If the depletion becomes more severe, that same person may go on to develop arthritis.

This could be compared to runners in a race. They would all begin at the same starting point, but as they run, someone may pull a hamstring, another may develop dehydration, and a third person may fall and break an arm. Some runners will tire very quickly, others will be able to run faster and farther before they tire. They are all in the same race and they all started at the same place, but the individual outcomes will be different based on a variety of individual variables.

Women and Autoimmune Disease

Women are more prone to develop autoimmune disease. Pregnancy and childbirth could be one reason why. During pregnancy, extra red blood cells are needed for you and your developing fetus. More vitamin B12 is required for pregnant women because it aids in the forming of red blood cells. In addition, birth defects associated with the spinal cord are increased if the mother has a vitamin B12 deficiency. The following information came from the National Institutes of Health (National Institutes of Health, 2009c):

"Women who don't get enough B12 may have a higher risk of giving birth to a baby with a potentially disabling or fatal birth defect. A new study shows that women with vitamin B12 deficiency in early pregnancy were up to five times more likely to have a child with neural tube defects, such as spina bifida, compared to women with high levels of vitamin B12."

Neural tube defects refer to a group of birth defects that affect the brain and spinal cord. Spinal cord degeneration has been found in fibromyalgia, MS, lupus, and myasthenia gravis. According to the National Institutes of

Health, subacute combined degeneration of the spinal cord is caused by a B12 deficiency. Vitamin B12 is necessary not only to prevent defects of the spinal cord, but also to maintain it.

"Vitamin B12 is essential for the functioning of the nervous system and for the production of red blood cells," says Duane Alexander, M.D., director of the National Institute of Child Health and Human Development which funded the study. "The results of the study suggest that women with low levels of B12 not only may risk health problems of their own, but also may increase the chance that their children may be born with a serious birth defect."

In a recent study from Denmark, researchers found that in the first year after conventional deliveries or cesarean sections, women had a 15 or 30 percent greater risk, respectively, of contracting autoimmune diseases such as lupus, rheumatoid arthritis, and multiple sclerosis (MSNBC, 2011).

The higher demand and ultimate depletion of vitamin B12 in pregnancy could lead to an increased risk for autoimmune disease. This could explain why women develop autoimmune diseases far more frequently than men. It is interesting that most autoimmune diseases occur in women during their childbearing years.

Sun and Chemical Sensitivity in Autoimmune Disease

Many autoimmune sufferers react negatively to chemicals and sun exposure. As part of the autoimmune process, sun sensitivity is due to a disorder called porphyria. Porphyria is caused by a deficiency of one of the components needed to make a substance in the body called heme.

Heme is a red pigment composed of iron linked to a chemical called protoporphyrin. Heme has many important functions in the body. Heme is found in the largest amounts in the blood and bone marrow in the form of hemoglobin within the red blood cells. Hemoglobin gives blood its red color and carries oxygen to every part of the body. As a component of proteins in the liver, heme has many functions, including breaking down hormones, drugs, and other chemicals.

The body makes heme mostly in the bone marrow and liver. The process of making heme is called the heme biosynthetic pathway. Each step of the process is controlled by one of eight enzymes. If any one of the eight enzymes is deficient, the pathway is disrupted. As a result, porphyrin or its chemical precursors, may build up in body tissues and cause illness (National Institutes of Health, 2008).

Porphyrin can accumulate in the skin and cause photosensitivity. Exposure to the sunlight may cause symptoms such as redness, rash, itching, burning, blistering, and swelling. Once triggered, an episode can escalate and cause even more toxic porphyrin to build up in the tissues, leading to even more serious illness.

The first component in the heme pathway is succinyl-CoA. Vitamin B12 serves as a cofactor for methylmalonyl-CoA mutase which converts methylmalonyl-CoA to succinyl-CoA. Therefore, a lack of vitamin B12 would lead to a failure in the entire heme pathway.

Once our body produces heme, it goes on to become an essential component of our bodies' first line of defense against chemicals and environmental pollutants; a powerful enzyme detoxification system called cytochrome P450.

The cytochrome P450 system detoxifies all sorts of different chemicals that we eat and breathe, including drugs, carcinogens formed in cooking, and poisonous compounds in plants (Guengerich, 2008). For instance, cytochrome P450 is the reason doctors tell you not to drink grapefruit juice when taking certain medications. Grapefruits contain a flavinol molecule that inhibits cytochrome P450 enzymes. This would slow down the detoxification of the drug and might cause it to have a stronger effect than intended.

The cytochrome P450 enzyme system also plays an essential role in hormone synthesis. It converts cholesterol into pregnenolone, which then gets converted into other hormones like estrogen, testosterone, cortisol, and DHEA. An inability to properly metabolize hormones due to a disruption in the cytochrome P450 enzyme system would account for the abnormal hormone levels found in autoimmune disease. For instance, in the study entitled "Endocrinological findings in patients with multiple sclerosis" half of the patients with multiple sclerosis were found to have decreased levels of estrogen.

The active site of cytochrome P450 contains a heme iron center, and therefore, cytochrome P450 enzymes are hemoproteins. A failure in the heme biosynthetic pathway would also result in a failure of the cytochrome P450 enzyme detoxification system.

In the following study, researchers discuss the association between Sjögren's syndrome and multiple chemical sensitivity (Migliore, 2006). The researchers believe that eventually further studies may reveal physiopathogenic mechanisms that both syndromes share.

Multiple Chemical Sensitivity Syndrome in Sjögren's Syndrome Patients: Casual Association or Related Diseases?

Migliore, A., E. Bizzi, U. Massafra, A. Capuano, L.S. Martin Martin. 2006. Arch Environ Occup Health 61(6):285-7.

Abstract: Multiple chemical sensitivity (MCS) is defined by multiple symptoms, affecting multiple organs, that wax and wane in response to varying chemical exposures at or below previously tolerated levels. Sjögren's syndrome (SS) is a common autoimmune disease affecting 3% of women aged over 55 years. Except for keratoconjunctivitis sicca (which is associated with SS not MCS), systemic features are common between the 2 diseases, leading to considerable morbidity and, occasionally, mortality. The authors report 3 cases of association between SS and MCS. Three women who were diagnosed with SS showed MCS symptoms and also were diagnosed with MCS. Further studies are needed to understand physiopathogenic mechanisms that eventually may be revealed as common to the 2 syndromes.

The Krebs Cycle

The Krebs cycle is a series of chemical reactions that occur within the matrix of the mitochondria. The main goal of the Krebs cycle is to produce energy. Essentially, the cycle involves converting the potential energy of nutrients into the readily available energy of adenosine triphosphate (ATP). The Krebs cycle is essential for the oxidative metabolism of glucose and other simple sugars. Thousands of times a second, one turn of the cycle turns a glucose fragment into carbon dioxide and water, just as if it had been ignited in a flame.

Just as in the heme biosynthetic pathway, succinyl-CoA is an important intermediate in the Krebs cycle. Vitamin B12 serves as a cofactor for the enzyme methylmalonyl-CoA mutase, which converts L-methylmalonyl-CoA into succinyl-CoA. Succinyl-CoA can then enter the Krebs cycle. Therefore, vitamin B12 is an essential component for the completion of the Krebs cycle. This is why vitamin B12 is called the "energy vitamin."

The body's main source of energy comes from the complete oxidation of glucose to carbon dioxide and water via the Krebs cycle. Fatigue, exhaustion, exercise intolerance, and brain fog are all directly related to impaired glucose metabolism.

Glucose is the only fuel normally used by brain cells. Because neurons cannot store glucose, they depend on the bloodstream to deliver a constant supply. Neurons, the cells that communicate with each other, have a high demand for energy because they're always in a state of metabolic activity. Even during sleep, neurons are still hard at work repairing and rebuilding their structural components. A lack of glucose would lead to mental confusion or lack of mental clarity. This is commonly known as "brain fog." Researchers at Mount Sinai School of Medicine have found that patients with Alzheimer's disease have lower glucose utilization in the brain than those with normal cognitive function (Varghese, 2011). They discovered that mice with impairment in brain cell energy production developed signs of Alzheimer's disease, such as cognitive defects and memory impairment.

Exercise intolerance is a common feature of autoimmune disease. In the research article "Chronic fatigue syndrome and mitochondrial dysfunction" researchers discuss the connection to exercise intolerance and impaired mitochondrial glucose metabolism (Myhill, 2009). They state, "What happens if some part of these cellular metabolic pathways goes wrong? If the mitochondrial source of energy is dysfunctional many disease symptoms may appear including the symptoms of CFS."

The researchers continue, "Suppose that the demand for ATP (adenosine triphosphate) is higher than the rate at which it can be recycled. This happens to athletes during the 100 meters sprint. The muscle cells go into anaerobic metabolism where each glucose molecule is converted into 2 molecules of lactic acid. This process is very inefficient (5.2% energy production compared to the 100% of complete oxidation) and can last for only a few minutes. The increased acidity leads to muscle pain. Also, when the concentration of ADP (adenosine diphosphate) in the cytosol increases and the ADP cannot be recycled quickly enough to ATP, another chemical reaction takes place. This becomes important if there is any mitochondrial dysfunction. Two molecules of ADP interact to produce one of ATP and one of AMP (adenosine monophosphate). The AMP cannot be recycled and thus half of the potential of ATP is lost. This takes some days to replenish and may account for the post-exertional malaise symptom experienced by patients." The researchers also stated that, "There is considerable evidence that mitochondrial dysfunction is present in some CFS patients. Muscle biopsies studied by electron microscopy have shown abnormal mitochondrial degeneration."

Multiple sclerosis patients also have impaired glucose metabolism. In the study "Cerebrospinal fluid evidence of increased extra-mitochondrial glucose metabolism implicates mitochondrial dysfunction in multiple sclerosis disease progression" the researchers stated that, "As extra-mitochondrial glucose metabolism increases with impaired mitochondrial metabolism of glucose, these findings implicate mitochondrial dysfunction in the pathogenesis of MS disease progression," (Regenold, 2008).

Impaired glucose metabolism also plays a major role in diabetes. Insulin secretion from the pancreatic islet cells requires ATP. The research article

"Interaction between Mitochondria and the Endoplasmic Reticulum: Implications for the Pathogenesis of Type 2 Diabetes Mellitus" states that, " Type 2 diabetes mellitus is characterized by impaired insulin secretion from pancreatic B-cells. In addition, insulin-responsive tissues, such as muscle, liver, and adipose tissue, exhibit insulin resistance. A number of findings suggest that both of these major features of type 2 diabetes are associated with mitochondrial dysfunction..." (Leem, 2012). The study found that "mitochondrial dysfunction in BAT (brown adipose tissue) appears to be linked to impaired thermogenesis and energy expenditure, contributing to the development of obesity and insulin resistance in adult humans."

Impaired glucose metabolism is a common occurrence in autoimmune disease, as is evidenced by the following studies:

1. Dalakas, M.C., J. Hatazawa, R.A. Brooks, G. Di Chiro. 1987. Lowered cerebral glucose utilization in amyotrophic lateral sclerosis. Ann Neurol 22(5):580-6.

2. Constant, E.L., A.G. de Volder, A. Ivanoiu, A. Bol, D. Labar, A. Seghers, G. Cosnard, J. Melin, C. Daumerie. 2001. Cerebral Blood Flow and Glucose Metabolism in Hypothyroidism: A Positron Emission Tomography Study. J Clin Endocrinol Metab 86(8):3864-70.

3. Carbotte, R.M., S.D. Denburg, J.A. Denburg, C. Nahmias, E.S. Garnett. 1992. Fluctuating cognitive abnormalities and cerebral glucose metabolism in neuropsychiatric systemic lupus erythematosus. J Neurol Neurosurg Psychiatry 55(11):1054-9.

The Krebs cycle is our source of vital energy. At times during my illness, it felt as though I had been literally "unplugged" from my power source; unable to climb a flight of stairs or even lift a telephone receiver at times. By providing our bodies with the nutrients they need, the Krebs cycle "furnace" will once again burn efficiently.

Endorphins and Enkephalins

Endorphins and enkephalins are the body's natural painkillers. The word "endorphin" is used generically to describe both classes of painkillers.

Endorphins are morphine-like substances that block pain signals in the spinal cord and brain stem. They do this by binding to the same receptor sites that pain signals use.

The body's goal in pain suppression is to allow the body to cope with pain while remaining focused, rather than allowing the perception of pain to overwhelm the system and cause panic and confusion. Endorphins are released by the brain and central nervous system when the brain perceives pain. They dull the sensation of pain and also help the individual cope with the emotional aspects of pain by changing the way the pain is perceived. Since endorphins can influence perception, they also play a role in memory formation and mood.

Studies show that autoimmune sufferers have lower levels of endorphins than normal. For example, the study entitled "Decreased immunoreactive beta-endorphin in mononuclear leucocytes from patients with chronic fatigue syndrome" found that endorphin levels were "significantly lower in chronic fatigue syndrome patients than in healthy subjects," (Conti, 1998). In fact, one of the drugs used to treat multiple sclerosis, fibromyalgia, and other autoimmune conditions is the opiate antagonist low dose naltrexone (LDN). It was initially approved by the FDA to treat heroin addiction. Low doses of naltrexone are thought to work by temporarily blocking the body's ability to release endorphins by binding to the same receptor sites. The body compensates by producing more endorphins than it typically would once the drug wears off. If you lack the ability to make endorphins though, this accelerated response could just further deplete your body's long term ability to produce endorphins.

The body makes two classes of endorphins, or enkephalins, from amino acids found in high protein foods. One form of enkephalin contains leucine, and the other contains methionine. The other amino acids found in both types of enkephalins are phenylalanine and tyrosine. We have shown that autoimmune sufferers lack these specific amino acids (Addington, 1999; Bazzichi, 2009).

It is ironic that an autoimmune sufferer's ability to deal with pain and suffering is severely handicapped, just when it is needed the most.

Human Growth Hormone

Human growth hormone (HGH) or somatropin is the most abundant hormone produced by the pituitary gland and the body's most important anti-aging hormone. HGH stimulates growth, cell reproduction, and regeneration. It is essential for normal muscle metabolism and repair. HGH also regulates the amount of sugar in the blood and promotes the breakdown of fat.

Chronic fatigue, fibromyalgia, lupus, and multiple sclerosis patients have all been found to have low levels of HGH. After failing to see an improvement in her patients with chronic fatigue syndrome after supplementation with HGH, Dr. Sarah Myhill, a CFS specialist stated, "My guess is that low levels of HGH is a symptom of CFS and correcting the underlying causes of CFS will result in HGH levels returning to normal," (Myhill, 2007b).

Many people believe that as we age the amount of HGH in our body decreases. In fact, the difference, generally, in growth hormone levels between adults and adolescents is not in the amount of HGH, but in its release. For instance, adequate amounts of blood protein levels will stimulate the release of HGH from the pituitary gland. The inability to digest proteins would result not only in a reduction of the amount of HGH, but also in the release of HGH from the pituitary. In the study entitled "Dietary protein restriction impairs both spontaneous and growth hormone-releasing factor-stimulated growth hormone release in the rat" researchers concluded that, "These results demonstrate that lack of dietary protein 1) blunts spontaneous pulsatile GH release, 2) attenuates GH responsiveness to GRF challenge, and 3) reduces pituitary GH content and size," (Harel, 1993).

Co-Infections: Parasites, Fungal Forms, and Bacteria

These are some of the more unpleasant side effects of having a pancreatic protease deficiency. Proteases are responsible for breaking down proteins into smaller amino acids. Proteases are also responsible for keeping the small intestine free from parasites (such as intestinal worms), yeast overgrowth, and bacteria. Parasites, fungal forms, and bacteria are proteins that additionally disguise themselves in a protein sheath that our bodies may view as normal. Proteases work by removing this protein shell. With the protective barrier down, your immune system can destroy the invading organism.

Oftentimes, autoimmune sufferers say their disease was preceded by a viral or bacterial infection. If you are bordering on a pancreatic enzyme deficiency and you contact a viral or bacterial infection, this would deplete your proteases as they would be needed to 'disarm' the invader.

Acid Reflux and Heartburn

If you frequently experience stomach problems, such as bloating, heartburn, gas, and indigestion, you are not alone. The antacid industry generates 24 billion dollars a year (McCormick, 2005). The problem, however, isn't too much stomach acid, it's not enough stomach acid. So, taking an antacid will actually make the problem worse.

Adequate production of stomach acid is required to close the muscular sphincter that relaxes and constricts to allow food to enter the stomach from the esophagus. When there is not enough stomach acid, this sphincter does not close, allowing what stomach acid there is in the stomach to regurgitate into the esophagus.

Low stomach acid is a condition called hypochlorhydria; and an estimated 47% of people in the U.S. have it (Hattemer, 2002). This is partially due to the increased use of antacids, which are marketed to the general public as a good source of calcium. A low level of hydrochloric acid can lead to chronic nutrient deficiencies, as the body's ability to absorb vitamins, minerals, and amino acids becomes handicapped. For efficient B12 digestion, acid is a necessity. One of the main functions of hydrochloric acid is to protect your body from germs. Once you lose that protection, your risk of infection from bacteria or viruses will rise.

Dr. Sarah Myhill, M.D., a UK-based ME/CFS/FM specialist, says that hypochlorhydria is especially common in those with fibromyalgia and chronic fatigue syndrome (Myhill, 2007a). She states, "The stomach requires an acid environment for several reasons. First, acid is required for digestion of protein. Second, acid is required for the stomach to empty properly. Acid is also required to sterilize the stomach and kill bacteria and yeast that may be ingested." She continues, "It is well known that the stomach must be acidic in order to absorb B12. Indeed, using a proton pump inhibitor such as Prilosec®, often prescribed for patients with heartburn or GERD, will reduce absorption of B12 to less than 1% of expected. Many people already suffer from borderline B12 deficiency– this is a difficult vitamin for the body to assimilate, but essential for normal biochemistry. Hypochlorhydria can lead to allergies. The reason for this is that if foods are poorly digested then large antigenically interesting molecules get into the lower gut, where if the immune system reacts against them, that can switch on allergy."

CFS specialist Paul Cheney, M.D., Ph.D., has also found that most CFS patients have low stomach acid (Sieverling, 2002). Dr. Cheney notes, "A UCLA study of 52 FM/CFS patients found Small Intestine Bacterial Overgrowths (SIBO) in ninety percent of the patients."

Hydrochloric acid works in the stomach to fight infection of the digestive system. Microorganisms such as bacteria, which are ingested in food and water, are destroyed in an adequately acidic environment. Sufficient hydrochloric acid is also necessary for adequate protein digestion. Hydrochloric acid is dually responsible for breaking the protein bonds when the protein enters the stomach and for the conversion of pepsinogen to pepsin; a digestive protease. Digestion then continues in the upper portion of the small intestine, where the pancreatic enzymes trypsin and chymotrypsin further break down the protein into amino acids.

Wouldn't it be great if there was a food that could raise stomach acid *if* it is too low, and lower stomach acid *if* it is too high? What about a food that could also give your pancreas the necessary enzymes it needs to properly break down proteins? In the last section of this book, we will tell you how to make acid reflux instantly disappear, and you will be *solving* the problem, not *masking* the symptoms.

Intrinsic Factor and B12

All B12 is initially manufactured only by micro-organisms, especially bacteria in soil and water, and to an extent, in animals' guts. Plants do not need it—so they have no mechanism to produce or store it—that is why they contain little to no B12. However, B12 is found in all animal products. In food, B12 is bound to protein, which is an arrangement unique to B12.

Assuring a good intake of vitamin B12, whatever the source, does not guarantee that it will be properly absorbed. In addition to a sufficient supply of HCl, a good supply of intrinsic factor is necessary for this vitamin to become available to the body. Intrinsic factor is a protein produced by cells in the stomach lining and is needed for the intestines to absorb vitamin B12 efficiently.

Intrinsic factor consists of tiny, innumerable open-ended protein capsules that bob around amidst the stomach acid (think Pac-Man). It is created by the stomach in the exact same shape and size required to fit a cobalamin molecule. These capsules randomly weave and bob around amid digesting food. When they bump into vitamin B12, they quickly trap it inside, snap open and shut, and transport it to the farthest end of the small intestine. *The small intestine is the only place in the gut where B12 can be absorbed.* Without intrinsic factor, most B12 would never reach its destination, because bacteria that line the intestine are hungry for this nutrient, and would intercept it. You can be starved for this nutrient even if it is richly supplied.

Making protein for intrinsic factor depends on a good supply of many different amino acids that are available primarily from animal sources. If you are not properly breaking down proteins, then you will not be able to produce intrinsic factor. Even if you take B12 in supplement form, your body will not properly absorb it.

CHAPTER 2 THE DISCOVERY

The Fibromyalgia Differential Diagnosis List – Don't Miss This One!

One of the members of an internet-based support group for people with autoimmune diseases recently posted a Fibromyalgia Differential List. There were 45 conditions and diseases on this list that share many of the same symptoms as fibromyalgia. This is not a complete list of every disease with the same symptoms, but the ones she felt were the most important to examine. The purpose of the list was to alert other members of the board to the possibility that they may actually have one of these other diseases and not fibromyalgia. Some of the other diseases listed were calcium deficiency, amyloidosis, adrenal gland dysfunction, Hashimoto's thyroiditis, mitochondrial dysfunction, vitamin toxicity or deficiency, diabetes, and Crohn's disease.

As I looked at the list for the first time, I realized that many of the conditions on the list were associated with the same enzyme-B12-protein pathway shared by the autoimmune diseases described in this book. I began to understand that the commonality of the symptoms was a clue that they all might originate from the same source.

To test my theory, I chose one of the diseases on the list that, on the surface, looked as if it could not possibly be connected to the autoimmune pathway. The disease was dysbarism, which can be seen in scuba divers. Webster's Dictionary gives the definition of dysbarism as, "A reaction to a sudden change in environmental pressure, such as rapid exposure to the lower atmospheric pressures of high altitudes. It is marked by symptoms similar to those of decompression sickness."

Webster's dictionary continues, "Nitrogen narcosis—Nitrogen comprises 79% of the air breathed by aerobic organisms, but at surface pressures it has no sedating effect. At greater depths, however, nitrogen affects the brain in precisely the same way as Nitrous oxide (also known as laughing gas)."

That part looked interesting. Here's what I discovered. According to www.wellness.com, "Nitrous oxide inactivates the cobalamin form of B12 by oxidation. Symptoms of B12 deficiency, including sensory neuropathy, myelopathy, and encephalopathy, can occur within days or weeks of exposure to nitrous oxide anesthesia in people with subclinical vitamin B deficiency. Symptoms are treated with high doses of vitamin B12, but recovery can be slow and incomplete," (Wellness.com, 2011).

The number one condition on the Fibromyalgia Differential List is Acid-Base Imbalances. About this condition, the member writes, "Acid-Base imbalances such as metabolic acidosis or alkalosis can be caused by bicarbonate deficit." The pancreas consists of bicarbonate, water, and enzymes. Bicarbonate secreted by the pancreas neutralizes acid and protects digestive enzymes.

The implications of this are astounding! While writing this book, I realized that the symptoms of a disease, not just an autoimmune label, indicate that it originates with a pancreatic enzyme deficiency. Anytime the enzyme-B12-protein pathway is disrupted, you will see symptoms of autoimmune disease.

The authors of this book would like to propose a new and more accurate term to describe the autoimmune diseases. Instead of naming them after their primary symptoms, i.e., lupus "marks of a wolf," rosacea "flushed blood vessels," myasthenia gravis "heavy muscles," we suggest that they be named after their cause, "Pancreatic Enzyme Deficiency Disease" (PEDD).

Pancreatic Enzyme Deficiency Disease (PEDD)

How can we determine if a disease originates with PEDD? Much the same way we know we have a cold, because we have the symptoms of a cold; runny nose, sore throat, fever etc. What are the symptoms of PEDD? Autonomic dysfunction, elevated homocysteine, low B12, elevated tumor necrosis factor, lack of essential amino acids, impaired glucose metabolism, and the inability to carry protein-bound calcium are all common symptoms of PEDD. If a disease originates with PEDD, then we should be able to trace every symptom and every valid scientific finding of the disease directly back to missing pancreatic enzymes. This is the PEDD pathway.

We would like to take seven diseases we haven't discussed thus far in depth to demonstrate how we can determine whether or not a disease originates with PEDD. The seven diseases are polycystic ovary syndrome, primary biliary cirrhosis, ankylosing spondylitis, Ménière's disease, interstitial cystitis, antiphospholipid antibody syndrome, and amyotrophic lateral sclerosis (ALS).

Polycystic Ovary Syndrome

Polycystic ovary syndrome (PCOS) is a disorder characterized by ovulatory dysfunction and polycystic ovaries. If PCOS is a symptom of PEDD, we should be able to connect it to the PEDD pathway. Since it is associated with autoimmune disease, this is our first indication that we will be able to. What are we looking for? A hormonal connection, since it involves the ovaries, an inflammation connection, since the ovaries are cystic, and autonomic dysfunction, since this is such a common feature of PEDD. Here we go. The following studies confirm we find what we are looking for:

1. Loverro, G., F. Lorusso, L. Mei, R. Depalo, G. Cormio, L. Selvaggi. 2002. The Plasma Homocysteine Levels are Increased in Polycystic Ovary Syndrome. Gynecol Obstet Invest 53(3):157-62

2. Paradisi, G., H.O. Steinberg, A. Hempfling, J. Cronin, G. Hook, M.K. Shepard, A.D. Baron. 2001. Polycystic Ovary Syndrome is Associated With Endothelial Dysfunction. Circulation 103(10):1410-5.

3. Gonzalez, F., K. Thusu, E. Abdel-Rahman, A. Prabhala, M. Tomani, P. Dandona. 1999. Elevated Serum Levels of Tumor Necrosis Factor Alpha in Women with Polycystic Ovary Syndrome. Metabolism 48(4):437-41.

4. Ghosh, S., S.N. Kabir, A. Pakrashi, S. Chatteriee, B. Chakravarty. 1993. Subclinical Hypothyroidism: A Determinant of Polycystic Ovary Syndrome. Horm Res 39(1-2):61-6.

5. Tekin, G., A. Tekin, E.B. Kiliçarslan, B. Haydardedeoğlu, T. Katircibaşi, T. Koçum, T. Erol, Y. Cölkesen, A.T. Sezgin, H. Müderrisoğlu. 2008. Altered Autonomic Neural Control of the Cardiovascular System in Patients With Polycystic Ovary Syndrome. Int J Cardiol 130(1):49-55.

Primary Biliary Cirrhosis

Primary biliary cirrhosis (PBC) is a liver disease that is characterized by a progressive destruction of the livers' small bile ducts as the result of chronic inflammation and scarring. PBC is an autoimmune disorder, and it has been associated with several other autoimmune disorders, including lupus, scleroderma, Sjögren's syndrome, and RA. Symptoms of PBC can vary from one person to another and can include chronically itching skin, fatigue, jaundice (yellowing of the skin and eyes), easy bruising, abdominal discomfort around the liver (upper right hand side of the abdomen), and bloated abdomen due to fluid build-up. Is PBC a symptom of PEDD? What should we look for? Since we know the scarring of the bile ducts is being driven by inflammation, we will look for elevated homocysteine and TNF. We will also look for autonomic dysfunction. And it wouldn't hurt to find evidence of a direct connection to PBC and the pancreas. The following research papers again provide confirmation of what we are looking for:

1. Biagini, M.R., A. Tozzi, R. Marcucci, R. Paniccia, S. Fedi, S. Milani, A. Gali, E. Ceni, M. Capanni, R. Manta, R. Abbate, C. Surrenti. 2006. Hyperhomocysteinemia and Hypercoagulability In Primary Biliary Cirrhosis. World J Gastroenterol 12(10):1607-12.

2. Neuman, M., P. Angulo, I. Malkiewicz, R. Jorgensen, N. Shear, E.R. Dickson, J. Haber, G. Katz, K. Lindor. 2002. Tumor Necrosis Factor-Alpha and Transforming Growth Factor-Beta Reflect Severity of Liver Damage in Primary Biliary Cirrhosis. J Gasteroenterol Hepatol 17(2):196-202.

3. Newton, J.L., A. Davidson, S. Kerr, N. Bhala, J. Pairman, J. Burt, D.E. Jones. 2007a. Autonomic Dysfunction in Primary Biliary Cirrhosis Correlates With Fatigue Severity. Eur J Gasteroenterol Hepatol 19(2):125-32.

4. Nishimori, I., M. Morita, J. Kino, M. Onodera, Y. Nakazawa, K. Okazaki, Y. Yamomoto, Y. Yamamoto. 1995. Pancreatic Involvement in Patients with Sjögren's Syndrome and Primary Biliary Cirrhosis. Int J Pancreatol 17(1):47-54.

Ankylosing Spondylitis

Ankylosing spondylitis is an arthritic disease that results in chronic inflammation of joints in the pelvis and spine. We know arthritis involves abnormal calcium deposits due to the inability to carry protein-bound calcium. The inflammation found in ankylosing spondylitis is our clue to look for elevated TNF and homocysteine. We have shown that rheumatoid arthritis patients have severe autonomic dysfunction, so we will check for a connection to this as well.

1. Başkan, B.M., F. Sivas, L.A. Aktekin, Y.P. Doğan, K. Ozoran, H. Bodur. 2009. Serum Homocysteine Level in Patients with Ankylosing Spondylitis. Rheumatol Int 29(12):1435-9.

2. Gorman, J.D., K.E. Sack, J.C. Davis. 2002. Treatment of Ankylosing Spondylitis by Inhibition of Tumor Necrosis Factor Alpha. New Engl J Med 346(18):1349-56.

3. Toussirot, E., M. Bahjaoui-Bouhaddi, J. Poncet, S. Cappelle, M. Henriet, D. Wending, J. Regnard. 1999. Abnormal Autonomic Cardiovascular Control in Ankylosing Spondylitis. Ann Rheum Dis 58(8):481-7.

Ménière's Disease

Ménière's disease is "a disorder of the membranous labyrinth of the inner ear that is marked by recurrent attacks of dizziness, tinnitus (ringing in the ears), and hearing loss," (Merriam-Webster, 2012). It was first described in 1861 by French physician Prosper Ménière, who identified the small fluid-filled canals of the ear (the labyrinth) as the vertigo-causing lesion site. Ménière's has a high association with autoimmune disease, as the first study shows, so we should be able to trace it back to PEDD. We will start with autonomic dysfunction, since we have learned that the autonomic nervous system controls the production of body fluids. The study on Ménière's and autonomic dysfunction below, states in the conclusion that "the cause of Ménière's disease is related to the existence of autonomic dysfunction on the affected side."

Since one of the neurotransmitters that regulates the autonomic nervous system is derived from B12 (acetylcholine comes from choline; B12 is necessary for the synthesis of choline), we will see if we can find evidence of a B12 deficiency in Ménière's disease.

Homocysteine follows low B12, so we will check for this as well. Elevated homocysteine could cause damage in a few different ways. In the research article "The Potential Role of Joint Injury and Eustachian Tube Dysfunction in the Genesis of Secondary Meniere's Disease" it states, "Eustachian tube dysfunction is a contributing feature." The eustachian tube is made of cartilage and bone. Cross-linking bands of collagen molecules are necessary to form the stable fibrils that compose cartilage. Homocysteine disrupts the intermolecular bonds of these fibrils. Inflammation and damage to the artery that supplies the cochlea (auditory portion of the inner ear), due to homocysteine, could also play a role. Arterial damage may even lead to thrombosis (obstruction of the artery due to a blood clot).

1. Gazquez, I. A. Aoro-Varela, I. Aran, S. Santos, A. Batuecas, G. Trinidad, H. Perez-Garrigues, C. Gonzalez-oller, L. Acosta, J.A. Lopez-Escamez. 2011. High Prevalence of Systemic Autoimmune Diseases in Patients With Ménière's Disease. PLoS One 6(10):e26759.

2. Uemura, T., M. Itoh, N. Kikuchi. 1980. Autonomic Dysfunction On the Affected Side in Ménière's Disease. Acta Otolaryngolaryngo 89(1-2):109-17.

3. Shemesh, Z., J. Attias, M. Ornan, N. Shapira, A. Shahar. 1993. Vitamin B12 Deficiency in Patients with Chronic-Tinnitus and Noise-Induced Hearing Loss. Am J Otolaryng 14(2):94-9.

4. Scaramella, J.G. 2003. Hyperhomocysteinemia and Left Internal Jugular Vein Thrombosis With Ménière's Symptom Complex. Ear Nose Throat J 82(11):856, 859-60, 865.

5. Gocer, C., U. Genc, A. Eryilmaz, A. Islam, S. Boynuegri, F. Bakir. 2009. Homocysteine, Folate and Vitamin B12 Concentrations in Middle Aged Adults Presenting With Sensorineural Hearing Impairment. J Int Adv Otol 5(3):340-4.

Interstitial Cystitis

We have already shown the central roles that tumor necrosis factor and homocysteine play in the pathogenesis of interstitial cystitis (IC).

In addition, another indication of the involvement of the pancreas in IC can be found in the study, entitled "Elevated urinary levels and urothelial expression of hepatocarcinoma-intestine-pancreas/pancreatitis-associated protein in patients with interstitial cystitis" (Makino, 2010). A pancreatitis-associated protein, called hepatocarcinoma-intestine-pancreas (HIP), was found to be "significantly higher" in IC patients. The study states that, "Urinary HIP levels were positively correlated with urinary frequency and bladder pain…"

Researchers have also found an abnormal peptide in IC patients, just as they have in patients with diabetes and rosacea. The peptide is called Antiproliferative Factor (APF), and it is a glycopeptide. In the study we discussed earlier, entitled "Hematologic and Urinary Excretion Anomalies in Patients with Chronic Fatigue Syndrome" we saw that chronic fatigue syndrome patients lack the amino acid asparagine (Niblett, 2007). The researchers stated that, "The reduction in the urinary output of asparagine in CFS patients noted in this study may be consistent with impaired protein synthesis, since asparagine is an important amino acid in protein structures, required for forming glycopeptides."

Studies also confirm the connection to IC and other autoimmune diseases. The following study, entitled "Physiopathologic relationship between interstitial cystitis and rheumatic, and chronic inflammatory diseases" determined that, "Based on clinical presentations, epidemiology, pathology and laboratory findings and treatment response, there is an important correlation among interstitial cystitis and rheumatic, autoimmune and chronic inflammatory diseases," (Lorenzo Gómez, 2004).

One final study entitled "The relationship between fibromyalgia and interstitial cystitis" concluded that, "These data suggest that IC and fibromyalgia have significant overlap in symptomatology, and that IC patients display diffusely increased nociception, as seen in fibromyalgia. Although central mechanisms have been suspected to contribute to the pathogenesis of fibromyalgia for some time, we speculate that these same mechanisms may be operative in IC, which has traditionally been felt to be a bladder disorder," (Clauw, 1997). The study also found increased nociception, or pain sensitivity, in fibromyalgia and IC patients when compared to healthy controls. We have demonstrated that this is due to the reduced levels of endorphins in autoimmune sufferers.

1. Makino, T., H. Kawashima, H. Konishi, T. Nakatani, H. Kiyama. 2010. Elevated urinary levels and urothelial expression of hepatocarcinoma-intestine-pancreas/pancreatitis-associated protein in patients with interstitial cystitis. Urology 75(4):933-7.

2. Keay, S.K., Z. Szekely, T.P. Conrads, T.D. Veenstra, J.J. Barchi Jr, C.O. Zhang, K.R. Koch, C.J. Michejda. 2004. An antiproliferative factor from interstitial cystitis patients is a frizzled 8 protein-related sialoglycopeptide. Proc Natl Acad Sci USA 101(32):11803-8.

3. Lorenzo Gómez, M.F., S. Gómez Castro. 2004. [Physiopathologic relationship between interstitial cystitis and rheumatic, autoimmune, and chronic inflammatory diseases]. Arch Esp Urol 57(1):25-34.

4. Clauw, D.J., M. Schmidt, D. Radulovic, A. Singer, P. Katz, J. Bresette. 1997. The relationship between fibromyalgia and interstitial cystitis. J Pschiatr Res 31(1):125-31.

Antiphospholipid Antibody Syndrome

Antiphospholipid Antibody Syndrome (APS) is an autoimmune disease characterized by blood clots, miscarriages, heart attacks, strokes, heart valve problems, and decreased levels of platelets. It has been estimated that nearly half of the people who have lupus also have APS. Given the symptoms of APS, we shouldn't have any trouble showing APS is linked to homocysteine. We will also check for inflammation's other partner in crime; tumor necrosis factor.

High homocysteine means low B12. White matter lesions are a sure sign of vitamin B12 deficiency. In the study entitled "Cognitive Deficits in Patients with Antiphospholipid Syndrome" researchers stated that, "Abnormal MRI findings in APS include single or multiple infarcts, white matter lesions, cortical atrophy, and focal hemorrhage," (Tektonidou, 2006).

Lack of vitamin B12 would also lead to impaired glucose metabolism. In the research article below on cerebral blood flow and glucose metabolism in APS, researchers concluded that "PET scans showed a considerable diffuse impairment of cortical glucose metabolism..." (Hilker, 2000).

1. Avivi, I., N. Lanir, R. Hoffman, B. Brenner. 2002. Hyperhomocysteinemia is common in patients with antiphospholipid syndrome and may contribute to expression of major thrombotic events. Blood Coagul Fibrin 13(2):169-72.

2. Swadzba, J., T. Iwaniec, J. Musial. 2011. Increased level of tumor necrosis factor-a in patients with antiphospholipid syndrome: marker not only of inflammation but also of the prothrombotic state. Rheumatol Int 31(3):307-13.

3. Tektonidou, M.G., N. Varsou, G. Kotoulas, A. Antoniou, H.M. Moutsopoulos. 2006. Cognitive Deficits in Patients With Antiphospholipid Syndrome. Arch Intern Med 166:2278-84.

4. Hilker, R., A. Thiel, C. Geisen, J. Rudolf. 2000. Cerebral blood flow and glucose metabolism in multi infarct-dementia related to primary antiphospholipid antibody syndrome. Lupus 9(4):311-6.

Amyotrophic Lateral Sclerosis (ALS)

ALS, otherwise known as Lou Gehrig's disease, is a motor neuron disease that rapidly degenerates nerve cells that control voluntary (and sometimes certain involuntary) muscles. Since ALS involves neurons, the first thing we will do is look for myelin damage due to lack of B12. We find what we are looking for in the study entitled "White matter injury in amyotrophic lateral sclerosis" (Rafalowska, 1996). Extensive white matter damage was discovered upon microscopic examination of six brains and spinal cords of patients deceased of ALS.

Lack of B12 could also lead to autonomic dysfunction. The following study involving autonomic impairment in ALS found a "wide range" of autonomic involvement (Baltadzhieva, 2005).

Next we look for elevated homocysteine. Our first study on ALS and homocysteine concluded that, "Plasma homocysteine levels were significantly increased in patients with ALS compared with healthy controls. ALS cases with shorter time to diagnosis presented high homocysteine levels, suggesting that higher homocysteine may be linked to faster progression of the disease," (Zoccolella, 2008).

An additional homocysteine study states, "In conclusion, several types of evidence show that accumulation of homocysteine may increase the risk and progression of motoneuronal degeneration," (Zoccolella, 2010).

We need to see if tumor necrosis factor is involved as well. Indeed, we find a connection. The study entitled "Pilot-Study of Thalidomide in Amyotrophic Lateral Sclerosis" states that, "Proinflammatory cytokines, such as tumor necrosis factor, are robustly upregulated in ALS."

1. Rafalowska, J., D. Dziewulska. 1996. White Matter Injury in Amyotrophic Lateral Sclerosis (ALS). Folia Neuropathol 34(2):87-91.

2. Baltadzhieva, R., T. Gurevich, A.D. Korczyn. 2005. Autonomic Impairment in Amyotrophic Lateral Sclerosis. Curr Opin Neurol 18(5):487-93.

3. Zoccolella, S., I.L. Simone, P. Lamberti, V. Samarelli, R. Tortelli, L. Serlenga, G. Logroscino. 2008. Elevated Plasma Homocysteine Levels in Patients With Amyotrophic Lateral Sclerosis. Neurology 70(3):222-5.

4. Zoccolella, S., C. Bendotti, E. Beghi, G. Logroscino. 2010. Homocysteine Levels and Amyotrophic Lateral Sclerosis: A Possible Link. Amyotroph Lateral Scler 11(1-2):140-7.

ALS patients are also deficient in the same essential amino acids we have found lacking in chronic fatigue syndrome and fibromyalgia. The study entitled "Plasma amino acids percentages in amyotrophic lateral sclerosis patients" found that ALS patients had significantly lower percentages of plasma tyrosine (which is derived from phenylalanine), valine, methionine, leucine, and isoleucine (Iłzecka, 2003).

These essential amino acids are derived from high protein foods. Lupus sufferers were found to lack the very enzyme necessary to break down dietary proteins into amino acids; DNase 1. MS patients also had significantly reduced levels of phenylalanine and tryptophan in their cerebrospinal fluid. They also lack noradrenaline, which is derived from phenylalanine. The lack of phenylalanine in fibromyalgia led to the lack of dopamine, which was discovered by Dr. Wood. Without phenylalanine, you would not be able to make either of your thyroid hormones or your adrenal hormones. You would also not be able to regulate your autonomic nervous system, since you would be lacking adrenaline, which is one of the regulatory neurotransmitters.

The lack of these essential amino acids leads to many of the symptoms found in autoimmune conditions. In turn, these symptoms lead us to the cause; pancreatic enzyme deficiency disease (PEDD).

CHAPTER 2 **THE DISCOVERY**

Summarizing the "Emerging Theory
About the Origins of Autoimmunity"

Studies from around the world have given us the scientific evidence to identify the cause of autoimmune disease. *Simply put, it all starts with the inability of your body to break down dietary proteins because you lack pancreatic enzymes.* It doesn't matter how your body is deprived of these essential pancreatic enzymes, the results will be the same. In the genetic disease Fabry, the deficiency in pancreatic enzymes results in the same symptoms any autoimmune sufferer would experience. When these essential enzymes were removed in mice, they too developed autoimmune symptoms. When prisoners of war became malnourished and subsequently became deficient in B12, they developed myasthenia gravis. Vegetarianism in India has caused much of the population to become deficient in B12, because B12 is only found in animal proteins. As a result, they lead the world in diabetes and heart disease. In the U.S., along with other nations with Western diets, we do not eat enough foods that contain vital enzymes and beneficial bacteria. This results in our body's inability to digest the same proteins that Indians do not eat. The consequences, however, are the same.

As the FM differential list demonstrated, the symptoms of autoimmune disease will arise anytime something interferes with your body's ability to break down proteins into amino acids and release B12. This happens each and every time with the same result, no matter how the deficiency came about, as was demonstrated with dysbarism.

Just recently, prominent researchers have begun to identify the abnormal proteins that are a result of these missing enzymes (as was found with the abnormal peptides discovered in diabetes and rosacea). These scientists believe that abnormal peptides are the trigger for autoimmune disease and that their findings support an "emerging theory about the origins of autoimmunity."

The recent spinal tap studies are also indisputable proof of the connection to pancreatic enzymes and the symptoms manifested in autoimmune disease. The lack of pancreatic proteases accounts for each and every symptom of autoimmune disease. The evidence clearly demonstrates the immune system is only targeting what it does not recognize, which are improperly broken down proteins and DNA, improperly folded proteins (amyloids), and peptides with missing amino acids. Since these diseases are the result of this deficiency, it would be logical to identify them with their cause. Pancreatic Enzyme Deficiency Disease is the reason you are sick. The evidence is overwhelming. Science and common sense have joined together to solve the mystery of autoimmune disease.

In the next section, we will show you how to replace these missing enzymes and restore the function of your entire gastrointestinal tract. You will be able to accomplish this with a simple, and yet powerful, healing diet.

Chapter 3 THE RECOVERY

Food as Medicine

"The doctor of the future will give no medicine, but will interest her or his patients in the care of the human frame, in a proper diet, and in the cause and prevention of disease."

-Thomas A. Edison, US inventor (1847–1931)

I already knew in my endeavors to eat as healthy as I could, that I needed to be eating organically. Since I was not a gardener at the time and was living in a small town, I was somewhat limited in the foods that I could get locally. I began ordering some items from a mail-order company in California that specializes in organic foods. I read on their website about a raw sauerkraut they carried that was having a positive effect on stomach issues. It was flying off the shelves at local farmers' markets. Since I had decided to focus on my stomach to heal my facial rash, I knew this was something I needed to try.

I received my first jar and started eating it a few times a day. On the third day, I thought I noticed some improvement in my lupus rash and was asking everyone, "Does it look better to you?"

"Don't get your hopes up," my husband said. Too late. I had been living with this rash for ten years and had tried everything from laser treatments to walking around with oatmeal on my face.

As I continued to eat the sauerkraut, the rash noticeably improved a little each day. After ten days, the rash was completely gone! Raw sauerkraut contains enormous amounts of enzymes and I knew that these enzymes were a key factor in clearing my rash. At that time, however, I didn't make the connection that the enzymes in fermented cabbage were also present elsewhere. Continuing to eat the sauerkraut led to an improvement in all of my lupus symptoms.

I no longer have allergies or sensitivities to foods, or anything else. I knew that the enzyme-rich sauerkraut, in conjunction with other lifestyle and diet modifications, was responsible for that. I realize now, that no matter how healthfully I ate, I would never get well unless I replaced my body's lost enzymes. But even though I was no longer sick, and my blood work was now normal, I was still left with fatigue. It wasn't the bone crushing fatigue I had felt with lupus, and not the fatigue where you don't have enough energy to wash your hair, but I was still tired. I didn't want to feel tired anymore. I wanted to feel healthy, strong, and alive. I wanted boundless energy, but I wasn't there yet. It has only been recently that I put together the B12 and protein connection.

To confirm my theory, I went to the doctor for a blood panel. I specifically asked to have my B12 checked. When the nurse called with the results, she said, "Your blood work is completely normal, except for two things. Your B12 is very low, it is 117. Also, your cholesterol is high, it's 278." She continued, "You need B12 shots and you need to change your diet. You should really cut back on animal products."

I responded, "Where do you get B12?"

She said, "I don't know."

I told her, "I do. You only get B12 from animal products. How could my B12 be so low, if I am eating too many animal products?"

"I'm not sure," she said.

A B12 level of 117 pg/mL is scary low. If you fall under 100 pg/mL, you can experience convulsions and permanent brain damage. As we have discussed before, in the United States 200 pg/mL is considered to be the lower limit, and is based on the level at which we find abnormalities in the blood. Other countries, however, use a lower limit of 500-550 pg/mL, which is based on mental changes, such as memory loss and dementia.

No wonder my energy level wasn't good. I initially related the high cholesterol to proteins not being broken down properly. I now realize that with such a low B12 level, my homocysteine level would rise and continue to damage my blood vessels. The cholesterol would be high, partly because it would be needed to repair the damage.

Initially, I ate the sauerkraut a few times a day. When my lupus symptoms started to subside, I thought the problem was fixed and in time my energy would return. So, I didn't explore fermented foods any further. I didn't know about kefir, real pickles, or the many other ways we can strengthen our digestive tracts. Eating sauerkraut once or twice a day is great, but it won't bring up a crushingly low B12 level. To do that, you need protein and you need to be able to properly digest it.

I refuse to take shortcuts on this. No B12 shots for me. I know too much about the amazingly complex system the body has to metabolize B12 and proteins. I will leave that up to my body. All I need to do is give it the raw materials it needs to make me healthy. Supplementing with B12 could be compared to baking a cake, but forgetting to add the flour. The cake would be in pretty bad shape right? Would you be able to dump a cup or two of flour on top of the finished cake to salvage it? No, because the flour must be added at the appropriate time and blended with the other ingredients. This, of course, is a simple analogy, but that's the point. The simple chemical process of baking a cake is nothing compared to the body's complex function. If it won't work to add ingredients to a cake after the fact, it certainly won't work to alter the body's complex absorption process of B12. That is why, time and time again, you read of people having high serum levels of B12, but low cellular levels, and suffering from the symptoms of B12 deficiency.

Research has also found that supplements "can interfere with B12 uptake, exacerbate the symptoms of B12 deficiency or even cause the creation of B12 analogs that increase the body's need for B12," (Fallon, 2005).

In addition, researchers in Norway found that heart-disease patients treated with a combination of folic acid and vitamin B12 had an increased risk of cancer and death, compared to patients who didn't receive the vitamins as treatment (Ebbing, 2009). The study, published in *The Journal of the American Medical Association*, followed more than 6,000 patients. Folic acid and B12 supplementation was associated with a 21% increased risk of cancer, a 38% increased risk for dying from the disease, and an 18% increase in deaths from all causes.

There are a growing number of studies that have suggested that supplemental folic acid and B12 can potentially speed up the progression of cancer in genetically predisposed individuals. *Folic acid* is not nature's *folate*. It is a synthetic form of folate, a vitamin naturally found in leafy greens and other fruits and vegetables. Evidently, your body knows the difference.

"We are concerned about folic acid supplementation actually promoting existing cancer," said Young-In Kim, Professor of Medicine and Nutritional Sciences at the University of Toronto and gastroenterologist at St. Michael's Hospital. He continues, "It's not hard for average Canadians to meet or even exceed the 0.8 milligram dose of folic acid given in the study." He is concerned about people who take supplements that typically contain 0.4 milligrams of folic acid. When you take into account the folic acid added to grain products, an individual could easily consume the dose used in the study.

The National Institutes of Health states, "Large amounts of folic acid can mask the damaging effects of vitamin B12 deficiency by correcting the megaloblastic anemia caused by vitamin B12 deficiency, without correcting the neurological damage that also occurs. Moreover, preliminary evidence suggests that high serum folate levels might not only mask vitamin B12 deficiency, but could also *exacerbate* the anemia and *worsen* the cognitive symptoms associated with vitamin B12 deficiency," (National Institutes of Health, 2010). You may need to rethink everything you thought you knew about fighting your disease. Your body can heal itself if you give it the raw materials it needs to function, in the form it was designed to use them in.

We would not want to do anything that could possibly cause us more harm. As we have discussed, sometimes taking supplements may not help us and could actually lead to an increased risk of disease.

In his book, *Nutrition and Athletic Performance*, Dr. Douglas Graham states, "Supplementation has proven to be an inadequate and incomplete method of supplying nutrients as scientists cannot match nature's refined balances. An estimated 90% of all nutrients are as yet undiscovered. Most nutrients are known to interact symbiotically with at least eight other nutrients. Considering this, the odds of healthfully supplying any nutrient in its necessary component package becomes nearly impossible. Why would we want to start adding isolated, synthetic nutrients into our bodies that could possibly increase our risk of disease, rather than eating whole foods?" (Graham, 2008).

Dr. Graham additionally states, "There has never been a successful attempt to keep an animal or human healthy, or even alive, on a diet composed of strictly nutritional supplements." If you can't stay healthy on supplements, how could you expect to overcome disease on them?

Low levels of vitamin D are also often found in autoimmune sufferers. Taking a supplement, however, has been shown to result in the same increased risk of disease as B12 supplementation. It does not address the underlying cause, which is the body's inability to carry protein-bound calcium. Calcium is necessary for vitamin D metabolism. You most likely have sufficient amounts of vitamin D, but your body is unable to metabolize it correctly.

An article from *ScienceDaily* entitled "Low Levels Of Vitamin D In Patients With Autoimmune Disease May Be Result, Not Cause Of The Disease" states that low levels of vitamin D in patients with autoimmune disease may be a result, rather than a cause of disease and that supplementing with vitamin D may actually exacerbate autoimmune disease (Autoimmunity

Research Foundation, 2009). Low levels of vitamin D would result if you were not able to carry protein-bound calcium, as we have seen in arthritis.

Authored by a team of researchers at the California-based non-profit Autoimmunity Research Foundation, their paper goes on to point out, "Molecular biologists have long known that the form of vitamin D, derived from supplements (such as D3), is a secosteroid rather than a vitamin. Only the sun can provide you with true vitamin D. Like corticosteroid medications, synthetic vitamin D may provide short-term relief by lowering inflammation, but may exacerbate disease symptoms over the long-term."

A form of vitamin D called cholecalciferol, also called vitamin D3 or calciol, is added to many foods as a supplement. It is also prescribed as a medication for people who are unable to maintain adequate levels of vitamin D. You might be surprised to learn though, that it is also commonly used as an ingredient in rodent poison. Here is an excerpt from the Merck Veterinary Manual on cholecalciferol:

"Cholecalciferol: Although this rodenticide was introduced with claims that it was less toxic to nontarget species than to rodents, clinical experience has shown that rodenticides containing cholecalciferol are a significant health threat to dogs and cats. Cholecalciferol produces hypercalcemia, which results in systemic calcification of soft tissue, leading to renal failure, cardiac abnormalities, hypertension, CNS depression, and GI upset," (Merck & Co., 2011).

The target organs for cholecalciferol toxicity in animals are the heart and kidneys. The heart and kidneys are also the target organs for cholecalciferol toxicity in humans. A report from the Institute of Medicine in 2010 states that, "Getting too much calcium from dietary supplements has been associated with kidney stones, while excessive vitamin D can damage the heart and kidneys. Some signals suggest there are greater risks of death and chronic disease associated with long-term high vitamin D intake," (Institute Of Medicine, 2010).

Here are some additional findings from the National Cancer Institute as reported by MSNBC News, "A National Cancer Institute study was the latest to report no cancer protection from vitamin D and the possibility of an increased risk of *pancreatic* cancer in people with the very highest levels," (MSNBC, 2010). If you address the probable cause of low vitamin D, which is the body's inability to digest dietary proteins and carry protein-bound calcium, you will not risk causing yourself further harm and you will get relief from disease symptoms. Also, we would not want to do anything that could damage the pancreas in any way.

That is how my "Fermented Foods Diet" was born. If you concentrate on eating whole fermented foods, this will allow you to properly digest proteins. Fermented foods will replenish vital enzymes and bacteria, and allow your body to obtain B12, essential amino acids, and other vital nutrients. Bringing your B12 level back up will take some time, but please, do it the only way that nature intended you to. Your entire GI tract will need to be restored. This work will be filled with purpose and unlimited benefits.

Chapter 3 THE RECOVERY

Healing Your Gut

The basis of healing your gut lies in being able to recognize a simple, but profound, fact. We cannot improve upon, nor duplicate nature. A healthy gut is home to thousands of species of beneficial bacteria that live along our digestive tract, from our mouths, to our stomachs, and throughout our intestines and colon. They help us digest our food, synthesize vitamins, and are vital for the proper functioning of our immune system. They work together synergistically and each species plays a vital and necessary role.

You have likely heard of lactobacillus and acidophilus, but what about the other *750 trillion* bacteria, yeast, and other microorganisms that are believed to inhabit a healthy person's body? These diverse micro-floras comprise three to five pounds of a person's body weight. They are all living, vital organisms that only nature can create and sustain. Man has not been able to even identify all of the species, let alone create them. These living bacteria don't come in a bottle or a pill. They come from food that is living, whole, complex, and in perfect balance.

You are sick because you have lost the beneficial bacteria that you were designed to have. What do you think would happen if all the bacteria in the world died? It would not be long before all life on earth ceased to exist. When we are sick, we often look to antibiotics, which kill bacteria, to become healthy again. 'Anti-biotic' means 'against life,' all life. They kill off all the bacteria in our gut, because they can't recognize the difference between the good bacteria and the bad. Only about five percent of our gut bacteria is pathogenic; the other 95% is beneficial and necessary for our survival. How do you fix that kind of destruction? By eating yogurt? By taking digestive enzymes? Remember, there are thousands of species of beneficial bacteria. How many strains does pasteurized yogurt contain? The pasteurization process killed off all the original bacteria. The few strains present when you purchase the yogurt were added back in. They will not restore your gut to its original condition. Thankfully, nature has provided us with foods that will. We will also need to avoid anything that can cause our GI tract further harm.

Chapter 3 THE RECOVERY

Things That Destroy Beneficial Gut Flora

Many of the foods we use in our daily lives, that we believe are healthy, are actually making us sick. Canola oil is one of these foods.

Canola Oil
One day, while preparing to make dinner, I went into my pantry to get some oil. I chose the canola oil I had recently purchased on a big city shopping trip to a Denver health food store. I didn't even make it through the pantry door. "Wait a minute," I thought, "what's a canola plant?" When I couldn't answer that question, I knew what I would be spending the rest of my day doing. What I discovered made me realize that I had been on autopilot. We can't assume that just because something is marketed as healthy, that it truly is. So, what *is* a canola plant? Not something you would plant in your garden, I'm sure. Canola oil comes from the rapeseed plant. The rapeseed plant is the same plant that gave us mustard gas in WWI. It is toxic. Even the insects won't eat it. It is also cheap and plentiful. Canadian scientists figured out how to extract the chemical that would kill you immediately, and then began to market the remainder as a health food; hence the name, 'canola oil', which is derived from 'Canadian oil'.

Producers of canola oil contribute five percent of their profits to the Canola Marketing Fund. I could go on and on about its structure and whether this oil, that can only be created in a laboratory, is something our bodies recognize. However, if it wasn't a food 100 years ago, it's not a food now. At least it shouldn't be.

There have been various animal studies done, including one in Japan, during which the animals who ingested canola oil actually died (Dewey, 1997). Canola oil depletes the body of vitamin E, which is absolutely essential to human health. The depletion of vitamin E results in increased dangerous free-radical activity. Free-radicals can cause widespread damage to your body.

Wonderful alternatives to canola oil, that are not inflammatory to your system, include:

- **Virgin coconut oil** – for cooking at high temperatures, as it maintains its stability even at high heat. It is a healthful source of saturated fat in the form of medium chain triglycerides (MCTs). One of these MCTs is lauric acid, which supports the immune system.

- **Extra virgin olive oil** – for cooking at low temperatures or making a healthy salad dressing.

- **Lard, tallow, and other animal fats from organic, grass-fed, pasture-raised animals** – are a great source of conjugated linoleic acid (CLA) and vitamin D. Saturated fats help with maintaining hormone balance, brain function, and vitamin absorption.

- **Organic grass-fed butter** – is another great source of CLA, which has been shown in studies to help prevent cancer and help muscle building and fat burning.

"Just Eat the Box"

One of the biggest mistakes most of us make when we start to improve our diets is to continue to eat boxed cereal. We might switch from sugary cereals to an organic loop or whole grain puff. My sister did it. Her kitchen shelves are lined with different brands of organic boxed cereal. But is it really healthy? My sister thinks so. "There's nothing wrong with those," she says. "They're organic and whole grain." Is she right? I tell her she'd be better off just eating the box. Here's why:

The following is an excerpt from an article called "Dirty Secrets of the Food Processing Industry" published on the Weston A. Price website.

Weston A. Price, www.westonaprice.org

Dry breakfast cereals are produced by a process called extrusion. Cereal makers first create a slurry (a thick suspension of solids in a liquid) of the grains and then put them in a machine called an extruder. The grains are then forced out of a little hole at high temperature and pressure. Depending on the shape of the hole, the grains are made into little O-shapes, flakes, animal shapes, or shreds (as in shredded wheat or Triscuits®) or they are puffed (as in puffed rice). A blade slices off each little flake or shape, which is then passed by a nozzle and sprayed with a coating of oil and sugar to seal off the cereal from the ravages of milk and give it a crunch.

This process of 'extrusion' destroys many of the nutrients that are present and renders the amino acids toxic to our bodies by denaturing the proteins.

In his book, *Fighting the Food Giants,* Paul Stitt cited a cereal company study in which four groups of rats were each given a different diet (Stitt, 1980). The first group received plain whole wheat, water, and synthetic vitamins and minerals. A second group received puffed wheat (an extruded cereal), water, and the same synthetic mix of vitamins and minerals. The third group was given only water, and the fourth group was given only water and the synthetic vitamins and minerals.

The rats that were part of the group that received the whole wheat lived for over a year on the diet. The rats that received the water and the vitamins lived about two months. The rats that were only given water lived for a month. The most surprising results came from the group given the puffed wheat. The rats that received the puffed wheat, vitamins, and water lived for only about two weeks. Upon autopsy, researchers found signs of insulin shock, with dysfunction of the pancreas, liver, kidneys, and the degeneration of nerves of the spine.

In an additional study, University of Michigan researchers separated their rats into three groups (Fallon, 2008). The first group received corn flakes and water; a second group received the cardboard box the cereal came in and water; and the control group received rat chow and water. The control group remained in good health during the experiment. The rats fed the corn flake box and water died of malnutrition. The rats given the corn flakes and water, however, died before the rats that just ate the box! Additionally, the rats given the corn flakes displayed schizophrenic behavior before they died; throwing fits, biting each other, and finally going into convulsions. See why I told my sister she'd be better off eating the box? It is so easy to make your own cereal and turn a harmful habit into a good one.

Oats for Breakfast (or anytime)
Our favorite morning breakfast cereal has to be oatmeal. Organic oatmeal is wonderful for you. Oatmeal has the amazing capacity to move through your body performing a myriad of health marvels. It lowers bad LDL cholesterol, slows digestion, and leads to a stabilization of blood glucose and insulin levels. Oatmeal also contains wonderful phytochemicals that can help prevent cancers, contribute to lower blood pressure, optimal weight, and healthy bowel function. If all these benefits weren't enough, it is also full of amino acids and essential vitamins.

Oatmeal is truly an amazing food. It is even more amazing when you don't cook it. Yes, that's right, don't cook it. Is picturing chewing a mouth full of dry oats making you thirsty? Don't worry, my whole family enjoys this recipe and every person I have ever shared this with says the same thing—"I love it!"

Not cooking the oats gives you a triple blast of enzymes. You just soak raw organic quick oats overnight in raw milk. Then in the morning, add a little more milk and fruit (my favorite is strawberries), drizzle with honey, and you're ready to eat.

QUICK OATS

- 1 cup of organic quick oats
- Add ½ cup of raw milk and squish down oats
- Drizzle with a little honey
- Cover and put in the fridge overnight
- In the morning, add milk to suit, organic fruit, and some honey

Trans Fats and Candle Wax. It's What's for Dinner.

When William Procter and James Gamble started their company, Procter & Gamble®, they hired a chemist, E.C. Kayster, to develop a process to hydrogenate cottonseed oil. This process would ensure the shortening would remain solid at normal storage temperatures. This was in 1911. The initial purpose was to create a cheaper substance to make candles, rather than the expensive animal fats which were in use at the time.

Electricity began to diminish the candle market, and since the product looked like lard, they began selling it as food. The product became known as Crisco®. Its name is derived from the initial sounds of "crystallized cottonseed oil." And so it began; 'trans fats' became a part of the American diet.

While there are beneficial trans-fats found in nature, such as conjugated linoleic acid (CLA), nature did not have a hand in making harmful trans fats. Harmful trans fats are man-made from artificially hydrogenated oils. They are produced when liquid vegetable oils are turned into solid fats through a process called hydrogenation. They have been a part of our diets now for over 100 years, but it has been just recently that we have begun to realize how deadly they are. There is no safe level.

Cities, towns, and even entire countries are banning trans fats. New York City was one of the first in the U.S. to ban the use of them in the cities' eateries. Montgomery County, Maryland, approved a ban on partially hydrogenated oils. They became the first county in the nation to restrict trans fats. California became the first state to ban trans fats in restaurants. They have been banned entirely in Denmark, Switzerland, and Austria. Yet, trans fats remain in over 60,000 food products.

Trans fats have been linked to depression, infertility, obesity, Alzheimer's disease, heart disease, liver dysfunction, cancer, reduced immune function, and diabetes.

Depression: Spanish researchers analyzed the diets of 12,059 people over a six year period and found those who ate the most trans fats had a 48% higher risk of depression than those who did not eat trans fats (Roan, 2011).

Infertility in Women: One 2007 study discovered that, "Each 2% increase in the intake of energy from trans fats, as opposed to that from carbohydrates, was associated with a 73% greater risk of ovulatory infertility...," (Chavarro, 2007). Trans fats pass from a pregnant woman's placenta to her unborn child. The unborn child's metabolism is adversely affected by trans fats in proportion to the amount consumed by the mother. Lactating mothers who consume substantial amounts of trans fats have less cream in their breast milk, since trans fats can lodge in the cellular spaces normally reserved for fatty acids. The cream is essential for maximum brain development of an infant. Increased dietary intake of trans fatty acids has also been associated with an increased risk of fetal loss.

Obesity: In June 2006, researchers at Wake Forest University reported after a six-year study, that calories from trans fats made laboratory monkeys fatter than calories from other forms of fat (Reed Business Information Ltd, 2006). In spite of efforts to prevent the monkeys from gaining weight by placing them on a low calorie diet, they gained it due to trans fat consumption.

Alzheimer's Disease: A study published in *Archives of Neurology* in February 2003, suggested that the intake of trans fat promotes the development of Alzheimer's disease (Morris, 2003).

C-reactive Protein (CRP): CRP is a known inflammation marker that, when elevated, predicts cardiovascular disease. A study of over 700 nurses showed that those in the highest quartile of trans fat consumption had blood levels of CRP that were 73% higher than those in the lowest quartile (Lopez-Garcia, 2005).

Liver Dysfunction: Trans fats are metabolized differently by the liver than other fats and interfere with delta-6 desaturase. Delta-6 desaturase is an enzyme needed to convert essential fatty acids to arachidonic acid and prostaglandins, both of which are important for cell function (Mahfouz, 1981).

Cancer: The European Prospective Investigation into Cancer and Nutrition suggests that the risk of breast cancer increases by 75%, due to increased intake of trans fat (Chajès, 2008).

Another popular trans fat is margarine. The manufacturing of this (fake) butter begins with cheap vegetable oils. These oils have already most likely been rendered harmful by the extraction process, which involves high temperatures and petrochemical solvents, such as benzene. One of the oils used comes from cottonseed. Cotton is not considered a food crop, so it can be highly sprayed with pesticides. In fact, it is the most highly sprayed crop in the world.

First, the oil is subjected to extremely high temperatures and pressure. Then, hydrogen is forced into a trans isomeric molecular structure to harden it. This process requires toxic substances, such as nickel oxide, which act as catalysts that enable the chemical change. The final product is a gray, smelly, greasy mass. Now it must be deodorized, again using high heat and chemical additives. This gray grease is then bleached white and then dyed yellow. Finally, artificial flavors are mixed in to make it taste like butter. Is it any wonder trans fats are linked to cancer?

Mankind has been consuming nature's fats, such as butter, lard, and coconut oil for thousands of years. Yet, heart disease only became common after 1920, when more people started to consume less expensive trans fats. Dr. Walter Willett, a professor of epidemiology and nutrition at Harvard Medical School, oversees the largest ongoing dietary study in America. Dr. Willett is a recognized authority on trans fats and has found that for every 4 to 5 grams of trans fat you eat, your risk of heart disease nearly doubles. To put that in perspective, some brands of microwave popcorn contain 14 grams of trans fat per bag. That is a big risk to take for a bag of popcorn.

Trans fats are not something to enjoy in moderation. As Tommy G. Thompson, Secretary of Health and Human Services for the U.S. Government stated during a trans fat press conference in 2003, "Trans fat is bad fat. The less trans fat people eat, the healthier they will be," (US Dept of Health and Human Services, 2003).

Trans fats have no business being in our food in the first place, so your goal should be to eliminate them entirely. There are many reasons an autoimmune sufferer should be very careful about not consuming them. Mary Enig, Ph.D., F.A.C.N. Director of the Nutritional Sciences Division

Enig Associates, Inc., states, "Because trans fatty acids disrupt cellular function, they affect many enzymes…," (tfX.org, 2004).

The distortion of cell membranes, as well as cell structures, is perhaps one of the greatest dangers of trans fats. When the cells are affected, every part of the body is affected. For example, the effect of trans fats on cell membranes makes them interfere with insulin receptors that are responsible for control of blood sugar. This could worsen diabetes.

In a healthy person, the cell membranes are made up of about 50% saturated fat. The saturated fats maintain the integrity of our cell membranes by keeping them stiff, yet flexible. This ensures that the cells function smoothly in assimilating nutrients, eliminating toxins, and keeping out pathogens. People who eat large amounts of trans fats have been found to have cell membranes that contain up to 20% trans fat (StopTransFats.com, 2007). Cells made up of trans fat, instead of saturated fat, become distorted and weak. Robert Erdmann, Ph.D., states that when the integrity of cell membranes is reduced, the lungs, digestive tract, and internal cells wind up "admitting allergens, undigested foods, viruses, and even potential carcinogens."

The human enzyme lipase, which is responsible for breaking down fats in our bodies, is ineffective against lipids in the trans configuration. This means that trans fats remain in the blood stream for a much longer period of time, are prone to arterial deposition, and subsequent plaque formation. *Once in your cell membrane, trans fats cannot be removed.*

If the integrity of the cells is badly damaged to the point where the cell membranes do not interact chemically as they should, the body's immune system may no longer recognize them. This could lead to an immune reaction. Been there, done that, right? Studies have shown that trans fats are incorporated into brain cell membranes and the myelin sheath. This could worsen the symptoms of autoimmune diseases like fibromyalgia and multiple sclerosis. They can also affect the brain in another way. Omega-3, an essential fatty acid, is vital for brain function. Trans fats are known to deplete the body's stores of omega-3, as well as its utilization.

An article published in *The Journal of Nutritional Biochemistry* states that trans fats can also cause endothelial dysfunction (Chen, 2011). As we have discussed, the endothelial cells are already under attack in the autoimmune sufferer. Since trans fats accumulate, the poisoning is cumulative. Furthermore, there are no immediate visible effects of consuming trans fats. As a result, the warning signs are missed until the damage is done years later.

On July 10, 2002, the U.S. Government's advisor on health policy, the Institute of Medicine at the National Academy of Sciences, reported that manufactured trans fats are an ingredient that *has no safe level for human consumption* (Food and Nutrition Board, Institute of Medicine of the National Academies, 2005). Dr. Jeffrey Aron, M.D., University of California, San Francisco professor of medicine, and one of the nation's leading experts on fatty acids, calls trans fats, "One of the worst hidden dangers in the food supply." The American Medical Association supports any state and federal efforts to ban the use of artificial trans fats in U.S. restaurants and bakeries. The FDA still allows trans fats in our food due to the enormous influence of the food and oil industries. Consequently, you must be responsible for safeguarding your own health.

In order to avoid trans fats, you will need to read the ingredient list on all food labels. Even if the food label states, "Trans Fat: 0 grams," and even if the product advertises zero grams on the front label, it may still contain trans fats. How is that possible? The FDA only requires food companies to list trans fat content if the food contains 0.5 grams or more of it per serving. What this means is, if a food contains 0.49 grams of trans fat in one serving, that food will have "Trans Fat: 0 grams" listed in its nutrition facts.

This FDA loophole can be very misleading to the consumer. First, few people ever eat one serving of anything. So, if someone happened to eat two servings of a food that contained 0.49 grams of trans fat per serving, they would have eaten just under one full gram of trans fat. Of course, anything can have 'zero' grams using this method by simply reducing the size of the serving.

A quote from the FDA's website explaining how a consumer can tell if a product contains trans fats states, "Consumers can know if a food contains trans fats by looking at the ingredient list on the food label. If the ingredient list includes the words, *"Shortening, Partially Hydrogenated Vegetable Oil,* or

Hydrogenated Vegetable Oil," the food contains trans fat," (U.S. Department of Health and Human Services, 2011).

The fats found in raw dairy and meat will help you heal, but trans fats, on the other hand, will bring your progress to a halt. Thomas Anderson, Ph.D., explains the difference, "It's important to understand that trans fats and saturated fats are completely different from one another and actually have opposite effects on health. The food industry's latest trick is to imply that both are 'bad' and should be avoided. This is a very dangerous deception, given that the fats in fresh meats and dairy food are important nutritionally. They lower the most significant risk factors for heart disease-including blood pressure, lipoprotein, and homocysteine. These foods also raise protective HDL and they reduce the risk for inflammatory related disorders, such as asthma and arthritis. The only fats we truly need to be worried about are the oils made into margarine and shortening and used for deep frying. These are added fats, they are not part of any natural food, and they are the only fats ever linked to any disease."

Products that typically contain trans fats include:

- crackers
- cake mixes
- granolas
- margarine
- candy bars
- cupcake and cake icings
- fried foods
- Cool Whip®
- potato chips
- hot chocolate mixes
- cookies
- pizza dough
- frozen snacks (pizza, pot pies, burritos, etc.)
- Crisco®
- fast food
- microwave popcorns
- soups
- ice cream
- packaged cheeses
- doughnuts

Medications

Going to your doctor for a prescription to solve an ailment may seem like the right way to find a cure. It's the way we have been taught, but many medications will only continue to damage your fragile digestive system, and will not allow you to heal. Healing you, however, may not be the number one priority of pharmaceutical companies.

You can read about this in Melody Peterson's book, *Our Daily Meds* (Peterson, 2008). Here is an excerpt: "In this profit-driven world of medicine, I did not often hear the executives talk of cures. Instead, they focused like honeybees circling a picnic cake on products for what they called the chronic disorders. These were the drugs that did not cure, but 'managed' disease as patients took them once a day for the rest of their lives."

These 'management medications' cause direct destruction of enzymes and beneficial bacteria, which will hinder a person's recovery. Some of these medications are:

- ACE inhibitors: including Accupril®, Aceon®, Altace®, Capoten®, Lexxel®, Lotensin®, Mavik®, Monopril®, Lisinopril®, Privinil®, Tarka®, and Univasc®- deplete zinc
- Acid reducers: such as Prevacid®, Prilosec®, Nexium®, and Aciplex®- deplete B12 and calcium
- Antibiotics: deplete beneficial bacteria, including lactobacillus, acidophilus, and bifidobacteria bifidu - deplete vitamins including B1, B2, B3, B6, B12, K, biotin, and inositol

Disease management is "Big Money Business"

Big Money Business

Peterson, M. -- former medical reporter for *The New York Times*, author of *Our Daily Meds*

Americans now spend over $200 billon a year on prescription drugs and this spending continues to increase by an average of 12 percent each year. Drugs are now the fastest growing part of the staggeringly-high American health care bill. Profits are soaring for drug companies, as the top 10 companies reported combined profits of $35.9 billion in 2002. This is more than all the rest of the 490 Fortune 500 companies put together! These same 10 companies spent $36 billion on advertising and marketing in 2002.

It seems the more they advertise, the more they rake in. But drugs have to be expensive, right? All that money for research and development has to come from somewhere. Don't believe it. In reality, in 2002 (the date of an extensive nonprofit investigation), only about 14 percent of Fortune 500 drug company revenues were applied toward research and development. Over 30 percent were devoted toward marketing and administration. Around 17 percent was received as profit. The Families USA, a nonprofit organization, reports the former CEO of Bristol-Meyers Squibb made $74,890,918 in 2001. This doesn't include his $76,095,611 of unexercised stock options. The chairman of Wyeth Pharmaceuticals made over $40 million, exclusive of an additional $40 million in stock options! Remember this when you wonder why your health insurance premiums continue to rise.

The drugs used to treat autoimmune conditions, almost without exception, damage the GI tract. The question is, to what extent? Prednisone is a common synthetic corticosteroid medication used in the management of autoimmune disease. According to www.drugs.com, common side effects of prednisone include insomnia, headaches, increased sweating, nervousness, and many others. One side effect stood out for me, and it is listed under minor side effects; "prednisone removes intestinal flora." What? That doesn't sound too minor to me!

Antibiotics

A study published in the February 17, 2004 edition of the *Journal of American Medical Association*, found a strong link between antibiotic use and breast cancer (Velicer, 2004). The authors found that women who took antibiotics for more than 500 days over an average period of 17 years had more than twice the risk of breast cancer. However, even women who had between one and 25 antibiotic prescriptions over an average of 17 years showed an increased risk. They were about 1.5 times more likely to be diagnosed with breast cancer than women who didn't take any antibiotics.

Anti-biotic means "against life." All life. Antibiotics disrupt and destroy many of the bacteria and flora of the gut that feed the immune system. Eighty percent of your immune system lies within your gastrointestinal tract (Institute of Health Sciences, 2010). That's right – 80%! So, it would make sense that if you destroy the very thing that your immune system needs to function, you would increase your risk of developing cancer or other diseases associated with compromised immunity.

One of the most important things you will need to do is not take any medication that will deplete B12 or damage your GI tract. And since most of them do, you may want to look for alternatives to conventional drugs. As always, never stop taking a pharmaceutical without help or consultation from your doctor.

My replacement has been herbs. When you have a mouse in the house, I think it is far better to set a mousetrap than to blow up the entire house to catch it. Herbs are the mousetrap. They will do the job of many pharmaceuticals without causing damage to your 'house.' In the resource section, I have provided the names of some of the best herbal companies in the country. They use whole herbs, organically grown and wild harvested, many of which they grow themselves. Herbs have been man's medicine for centuries. They are just medicinal foods, and your body will recognize them.

Here are two herbs that I have used to manage my own symptoms.

White Willow Bark: A Natural Pain Reliever

Long before we had aspirin, we had white willow bark. Ancient Egyptians used the bark of this tree for inflammation. The Greek physician and philosopher, Hippocrates, wrote about the use of white willow to ease aches and pains and reduce fevers. In China, white willow bark has been used as a treatment for pain and fever since 500 B.C. Native Americans used white willow bark for headaches, fever, sore muscles, and rheumatism.

Aspirin is an artificial derivative of white willow. Aspirin consists of just one of the many compounds naturally found in the whole bark—salicylic acid. It must be covered in buffers, because it is *acid*. Every time you take an aspirin, you bleed a teaspoon of blood from the lining of your stomach. If you don't think that is a big deal, rub a spoon against the back of your hand until it bleeds a teaspoon of blood. That is what your stomach lining looks like.

White willow bark, on the other hand, has none of the side effects of aspirin. It contains tannins, and the bark is actually good for your stomach.

It has also been shown to be more effective in relieving pain than aspirin and for longer periods of time. I use the whole, organic powdered bark in capsule form anytime I would use an aspirin.

Licorice Root: A Natural Anti-Inflammatory

The second herb I have used to manage the inflammatory symptoms associated with lupus is licorice root. Here is an herb that is 50 times sweeter than sugar. It is one of the most widely used medicinal herbs worldwide and is the single most used herb in Chinese medicine. An estimated 5,000 Chinese herbal formulas use it as a sweetener and to harmonize contrasting herbs. Its use dates back centuries. The Egyptians used it, as did Alexander the Great. In a recent survey of Western medical herbalists, it ranked as the tenth most important herb used in clinical practice.

In the treatment of autoimmune disease, this herb could play an important role. It acts on the adrenals, much the same way as corticosteroids. Except with one big difference, it has none of the side effects of steroids. Rather than harming the adrenals, it supports them. Rather than pushing them to exhaustion, it feeds them. It has actually been called, "Food for the Adrenals."

Licorice root is a potent anti-inflammatory. It is also anti-viral and antibacterial. Studies have shown it to have an extremely high success rate in the treatment of ulcers. It is not an immune booster, but rather an immunomodulator. If the immune system is overactive, it will bring it back into balance.

So, is there a downside? I could find no documented side effects from any study where the whole root, and not an extract, was used. An extract from an herb is not the same as the whole herb. Manufacturers often pick only what they think is the active ingredient, among many, in an herb. Many times, they haven't identified all the compounds, let alone what they are able to do. Even when extracts were used, side effects were minimal. They were generally associated with an increased risk of high blood pressure.

In a study conducted at the University of Tokyo, herbs were given to lupus patients who had kidney damage that was additionally aggravated by taking the standard anti-inflammatory drugs such as prednisone and azathioprin (Williams, 1999). The study found that approximately 25% of the patients stopped having relapses and were able to discontinue taking the drugs, once they began taking anti-inflammatory herbs. The herbs included bupleurum (which protects kidney cells) and licorice. These are examples of alternative anti-inflammatories that are very powerful, but without any of the horrible side-effects of the common autoimmune therapies in use today.

Licorice root is not to be taken if you are presently on steroids or any other medication for that matter. If you, at any point, would like to use it, then I would recommend consulting someone familiar with the use of licorice root. The government has placed licorice root on the GRAS list, standing for "Generally Recognized As Safe." I have used licorice root for many years. It has been a true lifesaver for me, and I am grateful that we have been blessed with such powerful, but gentle healers.

Chapter 3 THE RECOVERY

A Processed-Food Future

Lupus, RA, fibromyalgia, and other autoimmune diseases are rising rapidly. In the last few decades, the incidence of autoimmune diseases has tripled. Fifty million Americans are now affected. More women are affected by autoimmune disease than heart disease and breast cancer (Hyman, 2009). Our western diets are no longer based on whole, living, foods. They consist of processed foods laden with strange sounding chemicals and ingredients your body doesn't recognize and cannot utilize. At the very minimum, they will not cause you to get instantly ill, but they offer nothing your body can use to complete the startling array of metabolic processes required for you to stay alive and disease free.

Processed foods not only do not provide vital enzymes and bacteria, they strain and deplete the entire digestive tract. If you eat something that is completely devoid of vitality, your body will need to give up its stores of enzymes and energy to process it. The chemical residues in processed food will cause your liver and kidneys to work extra hard to protect your cells from the poisons they contain.

What you choose to put into your body, whether it is a food or medication, will have far reaching and profound effects on your recovery. Many people will read this book and think that switching to organic, raw, and grass-fed food is too expensive. The reasons we are sick are not entirely the food industry's fault. We, as consumers, want cheap food, and the food industry has been doing a great job of complying with these demands. However, we still pay for that choice, with higher insurance premiums, medical bills, medications, missed work days, and with our precious health and vitality.

Just as autoimmune disease is increasing, so is the earlier mortality of our children. Ours is the first generation where our children will not live as long as we do. If we fail to recognize the close connection between our food and our health, and don't start demanding better choices for us and our children, the future will only continue to grow dimmer.

Story of a 23-Year-Old: A Glimpse of the Future

Yesterday, a 23-year-old young man sat at my kitchen counter. He asked me if I knew how to get rid of arthritis. "Who has arthritis?" I asked.

"I do," he replied. He proceeded to tell me how stiff and painful his hands would often get. I told him it could be related to his diet. "What have you eaten today?" I asked. It was 5:00 p.m.

He said, "Well, I had some crackers for breakfast and I just had a cheeseburger and a pop."

"That could be your answer," I said. "Do you eat foods that contain enzymes?" I knew from the blank look on his face that he didn't know what I was talking about. I told him enzymes were found in foods like fruits, vegetables, raw milk, and kefir.

"I drink a lot of milk." he said.

I went to my refrigerator and took out a green smoothie (I will tell you about these later) that I hadn't blended yet. I pointed out the beautiful colors and the ginger and the kiwi that were loaded with enzymes. I blended it for him to try.

"Not bad." he said.

"If you continue to eat the way you are, your arthritis will only get worse," I told him. "You are 23; this shouldn't happen to you at 23. Not at any age really."

I plan to give him a copy of this book. He might not be quite ready to change his diet, but I'm sure the day will come.

Chapter 3 THE RECOVERY

Proteins

In order to recover from autoimmune disease, you will need to eat animal protein, and you will need to be able to digest it properly. You can't just go to Walmart®, however, and buy a steak for dinner. Your proteins will need to be free of antibiotics and hormones, and they must have been raised the way nature intended them to be. If the animal wasn't raised on pasture, then the eggs or meat will contain little to no vitamin B12. B12 is found in soil. You will be paying a little more for pure proteins, but it will be money well spent. This is medicine for your body. If you needed a drug to keep your heart pumping, you would not mind paying a little more for a drug that was free of contaminants. Not just any drug would do, and not just any protein will do.

As necessary as proteins are, if you can't properly digest them, you will do more harm than good. Initially, you should concentrate on healing your GI tract and restoring your pancreatic enzymes. When you feel your digestion is improved, you can start adding proteins. For most people this period will last a week to ten days. Always consume something fermented with proteins to aid in the digestion process. We will be discussing fermented foods in the next section.

Let's Start with Fish

Do you eat fish because you think it's healthy and is a rich source of vital omega-3s? How about salmon? Where does your salmon come from?

Would you be surprised to learn that farmed salmon is perhaps the most contaminated food on supermarket shelves? According to British government advisors, it is the *most toxic* food you can consume. In every batch they tested, the salmon contained at least three toxic chemicals: DDT, dieldrin, and hexachlorobenzene. Pollutants concentrate in farmed salmon because they are fed fish pellets and oils that are themselves contaminated.

"Farmed salmon is the worst of the worst of all foodstuffs tested for DDT, dieldrin, and other cancer-causing chemicals. It is a contaminated product," said Don Staniford, author of the article "Exposing the Salmon Industry," (Edwards, 2002).

And that pretty orange color? Where does it come from? It's a dye. Farmed salmon is gray. Wild salmon is orange because the salmon eat a natural diet of krill (tiny shrimp). The dye is in the pellets given to the salmon. It is called canthaxanthin and it has been linked to human eye defects and retinal damage. Don't be fooled by the term 'Atlantic Salmon.' That doesn't mean it came from the Atlantic Ocean. It is the breed of fish. In fact, that is the breed that is most often farmed.

For people with autoimmune disease, there is another issue. Farmed salmon are fed huge amounts of antibiotics. Antibiotics are needed to control the spread of infection in the high-density conditions of factory fish farming. In addition, the antibiotics we ingest in our foods from factory farming operations, as well as the antibiotics that go into our water supply, are believed to be a contributing factor to the growing antibiotic resistance problem in the U.S.

Fish can be healthy or extremely harmful. After learning how toxic fish can be, I began sourcing it carefully from Alaska. I eat wild salmon, black cod, and halibut. Most of my fish comes from the deepest, coldest parts of the waters around Alaska. Sadly, our streams, lakes, and oceans are no longer the safe, clean sources of food they once were. We need to be extremely cautious when sourcing our fish.

Chicken

Do you think it would be a good idea to eat arsenic? Most anyone would answer, "No!" It would poison you, right? In fact, the scientific definition of arsenic is, "A highly poisonous element having three allotropic forms, yellow, black, and grey. Arsenic and its compounds are used in insecticides, weed killers, and various alloys. Atomic number 33," (American Heritage Science Dictionary, 2005).

Arsenic and its compounds are especially potent poisons. To deliberately add it to any food meant for human consumption would be irresponsible. And yet, arsenic is added to animal feed, particularly in the U.S., as a method of disease prevention and growth stimulation. For example, roxarsone is an arsenic-containing compound that has been used as a broiler starter by about 70% of the broiler growers since 1995 (Jones, 2007). Broiler chickens are a type of chicken specifically raised for meat production. The Poison-Free Poultry Act of 2009 proposed to ban the use of roxarsone in swine and poultry production.

Researchers from the National Institutes of Health and the USDA's Food Safety Inspection Service looked at 5,000 broiler chicken samples and found alarmingly high levels of arsenic contamination (Taylor, 2004). The amount of arsenic found in the broiler chickens greatly exceeded the Environmental Protection Agency's (EPA) upper safety limit of arsenic allowed in drinking water. The level of arsenic in the chicken sampled was six to nine times that allowed by the EPA.

The animals Americans eat are so heavily infested with internal parasites that adding arsenic to the feed can result in a "stunning increase in growth rates," says Donald Herman, a former Environmental Protection Agency researcher who has studied this use of arsenic for a decade. "They [the poultry industry] have tried everything to refrain it from becoming public knowledge," he stated.

The poultry industry argues that the organic form of arsenic given to chickens isn't toxic. The researchers, however, found not only elevated levels of organic arsenic in chicken meat; they found elevated levels of the highly toxic, inorganic form typically used only in insecticides and weed killers. Inorganic arsenic is a human carcinogen linked to liver, lung, skin, kidney, bladder, and prostate cancers. It can also cause metabolic, neurological, cardiovascular, gastrointestinal, and immune system abnormalities. Arsenic is poison. Most poisons work by *specific inhibition of enzymes*. Commercial chicken is also heavily laden with antibiotics; another saboteur to your goal of restoring your gut flora. You can eat chicken; just make sure it is organic, pastured chicken.

Eggs

Not all eggs are created equal. Most people would naturally assume that if they purchased organic free range eggs, they would be making a healthy choice. I was one of those people. I used to buy organic free range eggs from my local supermarket. As I became more educated about the benefits of hens raised on pasture, and the dramatic increase in the egg's nutrition, I decided to do a little more research into the eggs I had been buying.

There was a phone number on the egg carton, so one day I called it. A nice sounding man answered the phone. I asked him if he could answer a few questions, since I had some health conditions and needed to be careful in my choice of eggs.

"Sure," he replied.

"To start with," I said, "How many chickens do you have?"

"60,000," he said.

I was shocked. "You have 60,000 chickens and they're all on pasture?"

"Oh, no, no," he answered. "The USDA definition of free range is they just have to have access to the out of doors. Our chickens are kept in big steel buildings with a concrete floor. We have two doors at the end of each building with a 5 by 5 ft. concrete paddock at either end. To be honest with you, they never go out there because we don't put food out there."

These chickens had never eaten a blade of grass in their lives. They had never taken a dust bath, which is their natural way to bathe. They had never taken a sun bath either, which would give their eggs natural vitamin D. They weren't in cages, but this was not a healthy environment for a chicken and these were not healthy eggs. If a chicken is never exposed to fresh air, sunlight, and soil, then their eggs will be lacking some very essential nutrients that we depend on for our health. The first of which would be vitamin B12.

Vitamin B12 comes from the soil, and animals need some of their food from the soil in order to ingest B12. In a natural environment, chickens scratch all day long in the soil for worms and bugs, and eat clover and other greens with soil particles attached. This is also important to keep in mind when you buy chicken to eat. Has it been truly pastured? If not, then the meat will not have B12 either. This, of course, is true of all land based animal proteins.

A study done by *Mother Earth News* found that eggs from hens raised on pasture may contain:

- 1/3 less cholesterol
- 1/4 less saturated fat
- 2/3 more vitamin A
- 2 times more omega-3 fatty acids
- 3 times more vitamin E
- 7 times more beta carotene

When I realized I would no longer be able to buy eggs from my local grocer, I began searching for an alternative local source. I wasn't very successful. I saw chickens that I was told were being pastured, which were actually being kept in dog runs with no grass whatsoever. I saw chickens with no feathers, huddled together in a totally dark building. I could find no one doing everything right. By that I mean, chickens being fed organic feed and allowed to roam freely on plenty of green grass. So, I got my own chickens. They are the most spoiled, pampered chickens on the planet, and they reward me with the most nutritious, delicious eggs I have ever tasted. At first, I was the only one in my neighborhood to have chickens, but after some of my neighbors met my chickens and tasted their eggs, they realized what they had been missing and got chickens of their own.

If eggs are going to be a part of your recovery, I would encourage you to be absolutely sure they come from truly pastured organic chickens. The only way to do this is to visit your source. Do the chickens look healthy? Are they being fed organic grains? What about cleanliness? Or, maybe you could just get your own chickens, as I did.

To start sourcing local eggs, you can go to farmers' markets and use resources like www.localharvest.org and www.eatwild.com. Sourcing food takes time in the beginning, but you will create your own little circle of friends who care about the food they are eating as much as you do.

Where's the Beef?

The ideal beef for you to choose would be organic, pasture raised, and pasture finished. All cows start out on pasture, but most cows end up in feedlots. Cows were designed to eat grasses, not grains. They have a four-chambered stomach to ferment the grasses as they move through their digestive system. When you consume beef from cows that have eaten grass, you raise your conjugated linoleic acids (CLAs) or omega-3s. CLAs are potent inflammation fighters. When you eat beef that was fed an unnatural diet of grains, you will raise your omega-6 fatty acids, which in fact, promote inflammation.

The result of animals fed unnatural diets is that they get sick, and they do so almost immediately. To keep them alive until they are fat enough to slaughter, they are fed massive amounts of antibiotics. The Centers for Disease Control and Prevention (CDC) estimates that 50 million pounds of antibiotics are produced each year in the U.S., and about 40% of those antibiotics are used in livestock. Nearly 80% of farm animals receive sub-therapeutic levels of antibiotics in their feed, at least part of the time.

In addition to the huge amounts of antibiotics, they are fed a 'hormone' cocktail. Today, farmers routinely use six types of sex hormones. Testosterone, progesterone, and oestradiol-17 beta, are the 'natural' sex hormones. Trembolone acetate, zeranol, and melengestrol acetate are the synthetic sex hormones. Like the steroids used by bodybuilders, these substances increase muscle and fat growth, making each cow heavier by about 50 pounds. They also make the animals grow faster, which allows them to be taken to market more quickly. Most of us would never take hormones without thoughtful consideration of the ramifications to our health. So why do many of us thoughtlessly eat these same hormones in the meat we consume?

This is not the whole story of beef, but for the purposes of your recovery, we will stop here and address what is relevant. Lack of antibiotics and hormones, high levels of omega-3s, and vitamin B12 are your very specific reasons to choose organic, pasture raised and finished beef.

Processed Meats

Consuming processed meats (hot dogs, sausage, bacon, lunch meats, etc.) can increase the risk of *pancreatic cancer* by a whopping 6,700%, according to a study conducted at the University of Hawaii (Nöthlings, 2005). This study followed 200,000 men and women for seven years. Additionally, leukemia rates skyrocket by 700% when a diet includes hot dogs. The World Cancer Research Fund (WCRF) has recently concluded that no amount of processed meat is safe. A previous analysis by the WCRF found that eating just one sausage a day raises your risk of developing bowel cancer by 20%. Other studies have found that processed meats increase your risk of:

+ colon cancer by 50 %

+ bladder cancer by 59 %

+ stomach cancer by 38 %

The culprit in these meats is the sodium nitrite. Sodium nitrite is a precursor to highly carcinogenic nitrosamines. Nitrosamines are potent cancer-causing chemicals that accelerate the formation and growth of cancer cells throughout the body. We need to restore the function of the pancreas, not directly cause it harm. Cancer aside, there is no hot dog or bologna sandwich that is worth having an autoimmune disease.

Chapter 3 THE RECOVERY

Beverages

It is estimated that Americans get over 20% of their daily caloric intake from beverages. This significant percentage shows that what we drink is an important part of our overall diet and will have an impact on our recovery. We may not always make the best choices in our beverages, reaching for sodas, energy drinks, sugary coffees, etc. The beverages many of us drink need a makeover. The first and foremost is our water.

What's in our water?

Fluoride: aka Hydrofluoric Acid

Fluoride is the ingredient that is in your toothpaste and that the dentist uses when you get your teeth cleaned. Fluoride is also the chemical they are dumping in our water supply, which we are drinking by the gallons.

Fluoride is not an element found on the periodic table, but rather an industrial by-product of steel, cement, aluminum, phosphate, and nuclear weapons manufacturing. Instead of it being a horribly costly pollutant that needs to be disposed of properly, it has cleverly been turned into a multi-billion dollar a year industry. It is used to produce fluorocarbons and chlorofluorocarbons for freezers and air conditioners. Fluoride is also used in the manufacturing of computer screens, light bulbs, semiconductors, plastics, herbicides, and toothpaste. The Merck Index indicates that sodium fluoride is used primarily as a *rat and cockroach poison* and is also *the active ingredient in most toothpaste*.

Fluoride was believed, for a short time, to strengthen teeth. As a result, our government began adding it to our water supply to create strong healthy teeth in our children. However, for the last 50 years, study after study has shown that fluoride does not strengthen teeth, it actually does the opposite. Fluoride is so bioactive that it interferes with the reactions necessary for collagen production. The mineralization of collagen is what leads to bone production and strong teeth. By disrupting this reaction, fluoride has been linked to osteoporosis, fractures, calcium stones, and crystals in joints and organs. Fluoride also disrupts DNA, which can lead to premature aging and increased rates of cancer.

For someone suffering from an autoimmune disease, fluoride is extremely harmful. Fluoride directly attacks the body's enzymes by changing their shape. Enzymes act like a lock and a key, fitting together to carry out the thousands of cell reactions that our bodies need for health and survival. Once their shape is changed, they become ineffective and often dangerous. Fluoride intake is increasingly being linked to autoimmune disease.

The following abstract shows the association between the first outbreak of chronic fatigue syndrome and fluoride in the drinking water. It states, *"Fluoride is a potent enzyme poison due to its affinity towards trace minerals."*

From the Abstract Chronic Fatigue, Fluoride and Heavy Metals
Phelps, J.E. 2005.

The term "CFS" or Chronic Fatigue Syndrome made its national appearance in the mid 1980's with the investigations of Dr. Paul Cheney concerning sick persons in the area of Lake Tahoe. South Lake Tahoe has public water supplies from wells that have metal contamination, often associated with volcanic zones or mining. South Lake Tahoe water reports have specific caution for immune compromised persons because of these pollutants.

Cheney's patients were from an extinct volcanic zone with contaminates in well water. From the study of volcanology, we know volcanic zones have many of the toxic FLUORIDES and metal problems associated with mining.

Fluoride is a potent enzyme poison due to its affinity toward trace minerals.

The Center for Disease Control (CDC) has advised anyone with a compromised immune system to consult his or her physician before drinking tap water. Healthy Divas, an organization dedicated to educating individuals about autoimmune diseases, advises avoiding tap water altogether. "Fluoridation of municipal tap water is voluntary at the state or community level," states Kathy Browning, co-founder of Healthy Divas. "We can't comprehend why they still add fluoride. Since the 1950s, research has proven time and again that it is unsafe. We do know that when our clients eliminate fluoride, many of their symptoms are alleviated," (Whitaker, 2006).

The Clinical Toxicology of Commercial Products handbook says, "Fluoride is more poisonous than lead and just slightly less poisonous than arsenic," (Gleason, 1957).

In his book, *Fluoride the Aging Factor*, Dr. Yiamouyiannis included a quote from a Proctor & Gamble* executive, saying, "A seven-ounce tube of toothpaste, theoretically at least, contains enough fluoride to kill a small child," (Yiamouyiannis, 1986). If you check your toothpaste packaging, the FDA now requires a warning be printed on the label. The warning states, "If more than used for brushing is accidentally swallowed, get medical help or contact a Poison Control Center right away." *Call Poison Control if you swallow your toothpaste?* Interestingly enough, the portion you use to brush your teeth (approximately 0.25mg), contains the same amount of fluoride found in an average glass of tap water.

In addition to our water and toothpaste, there are numerous other sources of fluoride that we ingest. Several steroid preparations also contain fluoride, so it may be in many of the medications that people with autoimmune diseases take. Some pesticides contain fluoride too. After all, what kills rats and roaches would surely take out the pests that threaten our fruits and vegetables. Buying organic food is once again the obvious choice over fruits and vegetables that have been sprayed with pesticides.

How do we ingest fluoride?

- drinking water
- vegetables and fruit – fluoride contained in the pesticides and possibly the water with which they are watered
- toothpaste
- canned foods
- processed foods
- soft drinks
- beer

Additionally, a 1998 lab test done at Sequoia Analytical Labs showed very high concentrations of fluoride in the following (Jones, 1998):

- Dole Pineapple® canned
- Snapple®
- Coke Classic®
- Hansen's Soda®
- Minute Maid Orange Juice®
- Gerber Strawberry Juice® for babies
- Amstel Lite® beer
- Rice Dream® (rice milk)
- Sunny Delight® orange drink
- Pepsi®

Fluoride aside, you should not be consuming anything on the above list anyway. It is important to drastically decrease your intake of fluoride, as it can be a direct obstacle to restoring functioning enzymes to your system. Using home filtration systems, eliminating fluoridated beverages, and not using fluoridated toothpaste is a good place to start.

This may not be a good topic to bring up with your dentist, unless you want to get yelled at. I am used to it, but you might not be! Ditch the fluoride and get a brighter, fresher mouth in return by making your own toothpaste.

HOMEMADE TOOTHPOWDER

- ¼ teaspoon organic powdered clove
- ½ teaspoon organic dried spearmint leaf
- ½ teaspoon of organic dried peppermint leaf
- ¼ cup baking soda
- ½ teaspoon sea salt
- ½ teaspoon organic dried sage

Mix the above ingredients together in a blender or small food processor.

You know how when you shampoo your new carpet for the first time, it seems to get dirtier faster? That's because a sticky, tacky residue was left on the carpet from the soap, which attracts dirt. The same thing is true of your toothpaste. If you use sticky, tacky toothpaste, your teeth will just attract dirt and bacteria. This toothpowder leaves your teeth feeling clean, with no leftover residue. And the addition of the herbs provides powerful antibacterial and breath-freshening properties that only nature can provide.

Plus, you won't need to keep an emergency number handy, just in case you swallow some!

Chlorine

Chlorine is another chemical that is added to our water supply. Chlorine has been linked to cancer, heart disease, and the potential for miscarriage and birth defects. Prolonged exposure has also been shown to increase the risk of rectal and bladder cancers.

The U.S. EPA defines chlorine as "a pesticide designed to kill living organisms." Should we be drinking this? Chlorine is used to kill harmful bacteria that may make us ill, but killing our own good bacteria, cells, and tissues is definitely making us sick too.

Even more surprising is where we get most of our chlorine exposure. We should not be drinking it or swimming in it, but should we be showering in it? It is estimated that 2/3 of our exposure comes from showering and bathing. The warm water opens our pores and our skin acts like a sponge soaking it in. Additionally, we inhale it as a steam. It is important to use a filter on your shower head, as well as for your drinking water.

The chlorine gas we inhale goes directly into our bloodstream and must be filtered out through the digestive system and the kidneys, which often are already overburdened. It has also been linked to increased bronchitis and asthma in children, which has increased 300% in the last two decades. Chlorine is a known carcinogen, but it also readily combines with other chemicals, forming some of the most environmentally hazardous chemicals known.

A form of chlorine, called dioxin, is produced as a by-product of the dye process for many of the things in our lives that are white. This includes writing paper, toilet paper, paper towels, Styrofoam® cups, and the inside of our milk cartons. A study reported in *Science News* found that the dioxin used to dye the inside of milk cartons leached into the milk (Raloff, 1988). Additionally, when you drink hot liquids from dioxin bleached cups, it leaches into the beverage.

Dioxins are endocrine disrupters. Your endocrine system consists of your ovaries, testes, parathyroid, thymus, thyroid, adrenals, organ tissue, and pancreas. Dioxins can interrupt the chemical signal process and severely compromise one's health.

Coffee

I like coffee (a lot). And I don't feel guilty drinking it. It is a primary source of antioxidants in the American diet. Study after study proves it is healthy in moderate amounts. There is one thing I insist on though, it must be organic! Most of the coffee grown in the world is sprayed with pesticides and fungicides containing dangerous chemicals. These chemicals, such as chlordane, chlorpyrifos, DDT, disulfoton, endsulfan, and methyl parathion, are so toxic to humans and wildlife that some of them have been banned from use in the United States. Among the adverse health effects of such chemicals are death, nerve poisoning, cancer, liver cirrhosis, sexual dysfunction, and more. When you pour hot water over the beans, you release these chemicals into your morning cup. That's not coffee; that's a witch's brew, and that is no way to start your day.

Chamomile

I rarely drink plain water. As I write this, it is 10:00 p.m. on the dot and I am enjoying a cup of chamomile tea. Of course, it has water in it, but it is boosted with the health benefits of this powerful, but gentle herb. Chamomile tea should be on your beverage list for many reasons. It contains compounds that will soothe and heal a damaged GI tract. It is a wonderful sleep aid due to its calming and relaxing properties. It also reduces inflammation, relieves muscle spasms, and has antiviral and antibacterial benefits.

Recently, research has shown chamomile to be effective in fighting diabetes. In one study, after 21 days, diabetic rats that received chamomile had significantly lower blood glucose levels than rats that did not.

To make my tea though, I didn't just open a box, put a tea bag in hot water, and call it a day. Here's why. Often, to get the tea in the bag, the herb is nearly powdered. This creates fissures, or cuts, on the surface of the herb. This is also true of other herbs in tea bags. These fissures immediately start to oxidize because they are now exposed to the air. They begin to lose flavor and beneficial health properties. When you are using an herb for its medicinal properties, it should be as fresh and potent as possible. To reap all of the benefits tea has to offer, I use organic loose leaf tea and brew it in a tea pot with a strainer. Remember, they are just foods. You wouldn't shred an apple weeks or months before you were ready to eat it, would you?

There is another, and perhaps even greater, concern. Does your tea bag look like a white pillow? Is it bright white with no string stapled to it? Then it has most likely been heat sealed with a potent carcinogen called polyvinyl chloride. It is white because it has been bleached with another potent carcinogen called dioxin. Both of these chemicals are heat released and water soluble. Do you know what that means? When you add this bag to a cup of hot water, you are drinking two of the most dangerous chemicals on this planet.

I ordered some bath herbs once from an herbalist who had taken great care in the growing and harvesting of the herbs, so I was quite surprised when I received them and they were in the pillow tea bags. I called and asked her if she had used polyvinyl chloride to seal them and explained my concern. Even though I wasn't drinking it, I didn't want to take a bath in it either. She said, "It's funny you say that, I used my iron to seal them, and it gunked the iron up so badly, I can't use it for anything else!"

If you use tea bags at all, be sure they have a drawstring and the bag is not bleached white. It costs the tea company a fraction of a cent more to do it this way. I am grateful they value our well-being enough to do this.

I never drink tea made with tea bags, simply because it doesn't come close in quality and flavor to a tea made from the whole herb. Once you are shown how to do it, it is the simplest thing in the world.

MAKING A PROPER CUP OF CHAMOMILE TEA

- Bring 2 cups of water just to the boiling point
- Put 3 tablespoons organic whole chamomile flower in a tea pot (loose leaf tea). We use a tea pot with a strainer inside
- Add hot water and steep for 10 minutes or until desired strength
- Add honey if desired

Green Tea

I drink two cups of green tea daily. I drink it because I enjoy it and because it has direct benefits to autoimmune sufferers. Research has long supported the antioxidant benefits of green tea, but now a study done by the Medical College of Georgia has found a direct autoimmune benefit. The polyphenols in green tea suppress inflammation. In addition, the study group treated with green tea showed lower levels of autoantibodies. That's good news!

There are many other health benefits associated with drinking green tea. The antioxidants in green tea have been found to be over 100 times more effective in neutralizing free radicals than vitamin C and 25 times more powerful than vitamin E. These same antioxidants have been found to reduce cellular damage that could lead to cancer.

Another amazing property of green tea is that it is calming, and yet energizing at the same time. Only nature could accomplish that. There is also evidence that green tea can help you sleep because it contains an amino acid called L-theanine. L-theanine reduces levels of the stress hormones, cortisol and epinephrine, causing it to have a calming effect on the body. The L-theanine in green tea helps to prolong sleep, reduce stress, and improve mental clarity.

GREEN TEA RECIPE

- Bring 2 cups of water almost to the boiling point
- Add 2 tablespoons loose green tea leaves to tea pot
- Steep for 2 minutes and taste for desired strength

Chapter 3 THE RECOVERY

Non-Organic Foods

There is continuous debate over whether organic foods are really any better than non-organic foods. Are they worth the higher price tag that we pay? For the autoimmune sufferer, the answer is an unequivocal "yes." To make the point, I want to share with you the chemicals in one bag of non-organic popcorn.

List of chemicals found in non-organic popcorn popped in oil from the US FDA September 2003 Total Diet Study, page 12-13:

US Food and Drug Administration Total Diet Study – December 2006

Summary of pesticide analytical results in food from the Food and Drug Administration's Total Diet Study program summarized by residue. Information pertains to (representative purchasable products) collected between September 1991 and October 2003.

p-methaxychlor	Chloroform
diclorobenzene	Diazinon
methyl-pirimiphos	1,2,4-trimethylbezene
malthion	Syrene
chlordane	Trichicreethylene
benezene	Cis-permethrin
xylene	Trans-permethrin
Polychlorinated biphenyls	Ethylbenzene
1,11 trichloroethane	Trans-chlorclane
Toxaphene	Cis-chlordane
Chloropyrifos	Dieldrin
1,1,1,2, tetrachloroethane	linclane

Not long ago, I had a man named Jim come to me for advice about a liver condition he suffers with. I recommended some herbal teas and gave him some suggestions about his diet. I knew it would be an uphill battle on getting him to eat organic fruits and vegetables. When you suffer from a liver condition, eating organically is especially important because your liver is your detoxifying organ. He would nod his head in agreement when I would bring it up, but I knew I wasn't getting through to him.

One summer day, Jim stopped by while I was freezing some organic peaches for my winter smoothies. "Oh," he said, "I did the same thing this morning."

"Really," I said, knowing there were no organic peaches available in town at that moment.

"Where did you get them?"

"Safeway," he replied.

"Were they organic?" I asked.

"No," he smiled sheepishly.

"Do you know where they came from?" I asked.

"California, I think," he replied.

"Let me show you something." I went and retrieved my computer and set it on the kitchen counter. I brought up a government database on the amount of chemicals applied *per acre* for peaches in California (www.pesticideinfo.org). There were 50 listed. I then asked him to randomly pick a chemical from the list. We looked up the chemical on another government database. It said if you ingest the chemical, you should call a poison control center. At random, I have picked five of the pesticides, from the list of 50, to show what they are and what health risks they are associated with.

(Please see the list on the following page)

Common Pesticides Used on California Peaches and Their Health Risks:

Pesticide	Uses	Health Risks
1,3-Dichloropropene	Fumigant, Nematicide	-PAN Bad Actor* -Acute Toxicity -Carcinogen -GroundWater Contaminant
Ziram	Fungicide, Microbiocide, Dog and Cat Repellant	-PAN Bad Actor* -Possible Carcinogen -Moderate Acute Toxicity -Developmental or Reproductive Toxin -Suspected Endocrine Disruptor
Copper Sulfate (basic)	Fungicide, Algaecide, Molluscicide	-Moderate Acute Toxcity
Copper Hydroxide	Fungicide, Algaecide, Molluscicide	-Slight Acute Toxicity
Copper Oxide (ous)	Herbicide	-Moderate Acute Toxicity

PAN Bad Actors are chemicals that are one or more of the following: highly acutely toxic, cholinesterase inhibitor, known/probable carcinogen, known groundwater pollutant, or known reproductive or developmental toxicant.

He leaned back in his chair, paused, and then said, "I've been poisoning myself my entire life."

I knew, for the rest of his life, he would choose organic if he possibly could, and so should you. For autoimmune sufferers, it is essential to choose organic produce that does not contain chemicals that will destroy enzymes. Pesticides are poisons, and most poisons work by specific inhibition of enzymes.

Researchers are finding a link between exposure to pesticides and an increased risk of developing autoimmune diseases, such as rheumatoid arthritis. This press release from the American College of Rheumatology shows that researchers believe there is an increased risk in developing RA and lupus with exposure to insecticides.

RA and Lupus with increased exposure to insecticides. Spraying for bugs could increase autoimmune disease risk – Press Release

Latimer, E. 2009. *American College of Rheumatology.*

PHILADELPHIA – Insecticide exposure may increase the risk of developing two well-known autoimmune rheumatic diseases in post-menopausal women, according to research presented this week at the American College of Rheumatology Annual Scientific Meeting in Philadelphia, Pa.

Farming and agricultural pesticide exposure has been linked to the development of rheumatoid arthritis and lupus, but it is unclear whether pesticide exposure in other settings might also increase risk of disease. The researchers believe these findings suggest that exposure to insecticides may increase the risk of developing RA or lupus in the general population, not only in the farming environment.

Chapter 3 THE RECOVERY

Personal Care Products and Indoor Air Pollution

Autoimmune sufferers need to be especially careful about what they inhale and put on their skin. Many of the chemicals found in personal care products, dryer sheets, laundry detergents, air fresheners, and household cleaners are known carcinogens. The Environmental Working Group (EWG), a public interest research group and advocacy organization, has found that more than one-third of all personal care products contain at least one known carcinogen. The average woman is exposed to 126 such chemicals on a daily basis. Sixty-percent of everything we put on our skin is absorbed into our bloodstream, so we want to make sure to use products that are safe.

According to the Environmental Protection Agency (EPA), indoor pollution is one of the greatest health threats of our time. A five-year EPA study of over 600 households revealed that contaminant levels in the average home are up to 70 times higher than those found outdoors. Dryer sheets, synthetic fragrances, air fresheners, aerosol sprays, and perfumes are all contributing to this toxic indoor air pollution.

The EWG has an interactive product safety guide called Skin Deep at www.ewg.org that ranks over 15,000 name-brand products (Environmental Working Group, 2012). The products you choose to use in your home and personal care should have a rank of 0. There is no need to use a product if it is hazardous to any degree. There are many safe alternatives available.

Chapter 3 THE RECOVERY

Yeast And Gluten

There is a high correlation of gluten intolerance associated with autoimmune disease. Gluten is a protein and autoimmune sufferers are unable to break down proteins properly. This gluey protein is found in grains like barley, rye, and wheat. It can strip the villi (little fingers in the intestinal tract) causing malabsorption, which can cause all sorts of problems. There is also a connection to lack of vitamin B12 and gluten intolerance. An important function of B12 is repairing damaged, flattened microvilli. With sufficient B12 in the bloodstream, the intestinal cells and microvilli can rejuvenate.

How did the 'staff of life' become something we should be concerned about eating? Remember what Jesus said, "Man must not live by bread alone." As described in the Bible, visualize his disciples walking through wheat fields and plucking off the tops of the wheat stalks to eat. So, what has changed? Not just the wheat itself, but the way bread is made.

Our ancestors, and virtually all pre-industrialized peoples, soaked or fermented their grains before making them into porridge or breads, etc. Through scientific research, we are now able to understand why and how it all works. Simply stated, the sourdough process transforms or breaks down food components in flour into a simpler form that is more easily digested. A diet high in unfermented whole grains, particularly high-gluten grains like wheat, puts an enormous strain on the digestive system.

Why did we stop making bread the traditional way? Convenience and money are both factors. Sourdough yeast lives forever if you take care of it. Once you have it, and you can easily get some from a friend that bakes sourdough bread, you never have to buy it again. So, where's the money in that? Fleischmann's first engineered "yeast that would die" around the 1860s as a convenience. Sourdough yeast takes longer to rise. The changeover became complete in the 1980s, when instant yeast was introduced. Once again, we've traded health and flavor for convenience.

What about someone who is gluten intolerant or has celiac disease? Would they actually be able to consume fermented bread, with no toxic effects? The study entitled "Sourdough bread made from wheat and nontoxic flours and started with selected lactobacilli is tolerated in celiac sprue patients" showed that even someone with celiac disease can eat bread with no toxic effects, as long as the bread is properly fermented. In the study, sourdough bread was made from 30% wheat and a mixture of oat, millet, and buckwheat flours. The bread was fed to 17 patients with celiac disease with no negative consequences. However, when the same 17 patients were fed the bread make with baker's yeast, 13 patients showed "a marked alteration in intestinal permeability."

In an additional study entitled "Safety for patients with celiac disease of baked goods made of wheat flour hydrolyzed during food processing" celiac patients were fed a 60-day diet of baked goods made from wheat flour manufactured with sourdough lactobacilli and fungal proteases. They also experienced no ill effects.

For someone with autoimmune disease, eating bread that has not been fermented will place an added burden on your already weak digestion. However, if you can find (or bake yourself) an organic, whole wheat sourdough bread in your community, by all means, enjoy!

SOURDOUGH PANCAKE RECIPE

These pancakes are easy and delicious; don't let the use of sourdough intimidate you.

The night before, mix well (to incorporate some air) 1 cup of your sourdough starter with 1 ½ cups of organic whole wheat flour and 1 cup of warm water (85°-90°). Leave at warm room temperature (70°-85°) overnight, covered well with plastic wrap.

The next morning, return 1 cup of the starter mixture to the fridge.

Then mix the remaining 1 ½ cups of starter with:

1 egg, slightly beaten

1 Tablespoon of honey (or more if you like)

¾ Teaspoon of sea salt

½ teaspoon (generous) of baking soda

2 Tablespoons of milk

Try to have your ingredients at room temperature. This will help to make the pancakes more tender.

Bake on a 400° griddle. Enjoy!

Chapter 3 THE RECOVERY

The Foods That Will Bring You Back
"The Fermented Foods Diet"

Just as factory farming is now the norm, the way we eat seems normal. That is not the way it used to be. Chickens on the family farm were free to search for bugs, grass, clover, or worms, and eat whatever else they found interesting. They took their baths in the sun and the dirt. They absorbed the sunlight and their bones stayed strong. The eggs had bright yellow-orange yolks filled with omega-3 fatty acids and contained 40 times more beta-carotene than a modern egg. The chickens were happy and healthy.

Okay, so we didn't used to eat bugs and worms, but our ancestors did eat fermented foods with almost every meal. And I don't mean our ancestors like cavemen ancestors. I mean just 100 years ago. The cellars of most homes were filled with raw fermented sauerkraut and pickles to last the winter. They drank fermented apple cider made in the fall and raw milk, kefir, and yogurt that they made daily. They snacked on raw cheese filled with enzymes and good bacteria. Their root cellars were filled with enzyme-rich fruits and vegetables like raw carrots, apples, and cabbage. In the summer, they ate vegetables and fruits from their gardens. These foods provided beneficial enzymes in abundance. They ate proteins too, including eggs and pastured meats, like beef, pork, and chicken. Our ancestors had the enzymes from the fermented foods they were eating to break down these proteins. Today, our diets do not include any of these enzyme-rich foods. Therefore, we are unable to properly break down the proteins we consume.

Initially, I would recommend that you refrain from eating too much protein until you have repaired some of the damage to your GI tract and restored its ability to properly digest proteins. Otherwise, your immune system will continue to target them. For about a week or so, focus on the healing foods we discuss in this section. Always make sure to eat your proteins with fermented foods, such as raw organic sauerkraut, in order to properly break them down. Your B12 stores, however, are dangerously low and need to be addressed immediately. At first, your main source of B12 and protein should come from kefir (which we will discuss in the up-coming pages). The proteins are already predigested and you will have immediate access to B12.

When you eat animal proteins, always make sure you consume fermented vegetables with them (such as raw sauerkraut), in order to properly break them down. By eating fermented foods, you are aiding your body in the digestion process.

The enzymes in the foods we will share with you as part of the "Fermented Foods Diet" including kefir, the green smoothie, raw milk, raw cheese, raw sauerkraut, muesli, and pre-soaked nuts, will give you nutrition without any burden on your digestive tract. These foods come complete with their own digestive enzymes and your body will not need to give up its precious stores at this most critical time.

Raw Milk

One vital source of enzymes is raw milk that has not been pasteurized, ultra-pasteurized, or homogenized. Is there a difference between the milk we drink today and the milk of the past? Dairy products have been consumed for thousands of years and are mentioned in the Bible as beneficial foods. Before pasteurization, milk was consumed in its raw form, and still is by many cultures. Even prior to refrigeration, raw milk did not spoil. It soured naturally and was made into butter or cultured into products similar to cheese, cottage cheese, kefir, and yogurt.

Modern milk, however, is the number one allergic food in the country. It is linked to so many of the ailments that raw milk can help alleviate. These ailments include:

- diarrhea/cramps/bloating
- colic
- skin rashes and allergies
- tooth decay
- heart disease and atherosclerosis
- type I diabetes
- rheumatoid arthritis
- excessive mucus production
- rashes
- mood swings
- gastrointestinal bleeding
- iron deficiency/anemia
- osteoporosis
- ear infections
- cancer
- arthritis
- autism
- allergies
- depression

What has happened to turn one of the most nutritious, virtuous beverages given to mankind, into one of the most harmful? Your recovery will depend on you getting this one right. Raw milk is a vital, living food, and medicine for our bodies. Raw milk, from cows that have been raised on pasture, is full of enzymes, amino acids, immunoglobulins (antibodies), metal-binding proteins, vitamin binding proteins, several growth factors, and beneficial bacteria.

Raw milk contains over *60 known enzymes* that have far-reaching effects in the body. Several enzymes in raw milk, including amylase, phosphatases, and lipases, break down starches, lactose, fats, and phosphate compounds to make milk more digestible. Other enzymes, like catalase, lysozyme, and lactoperoxidase, help kill unwanted bacteria both in the milk and in our bodies. In fact, many people who are lactose intolerant, or even allergic to milk, experience no symptoms when they drink raw milk. This is because the enzymes are present to aid in digestion and assimilation of the key nutrients and minerals. One of these enzymes is lactase. Lactase is responsible for the digestion of lactose in milk. When milk is pasteurized, this enzyme is destroyed and people may experience 'lactose intolerance' as a result.

During pasteurization, the milk is forcefully heated to high temperatures in a process that resembles nothing it would be exposed to in nature. This heating kills all the enzymes. In fact, the death of the enzymes is how they determine the process was successful. When all the enzymes are dead, the pasteurization process is complete. One of the missing enzymes, phosphatase, is necessary for the assimilation of calcium. So, drinking pasteurized milk does little to nothing in terms of building strong teeth and bones. There are 59 other missing enzymes that were meant for equally important functions within the human body. Pasteurization also results in the loss and/or adulteration of vitamins A, D, and E. Up to 60% of these fat-soluble vitamins are lost. Vitamin C loss is upwards of 50%. *Vitamin B6 and B12 are completely destroyed.*

Lactoferrin is just one of the many proteins found in raw milk. Lactoferrin binds iron, contributing to increased absorption and assimilation. This protein is also said to have antibacterial activity against several species of bacteria that contribute to tooth decay. Conversely, pasteurized milk contributes to tooth decay and anemia, partially due to the lactoferrin being denatured and no longer able to perform its function.

The denaturing of proteins during the pasteurization process is of grave importance to the autoimmune sufferer. During pasteurization, proteins are deformed, denatured, and broken up in such a way that the body thinks they are foreign. The body will then mount an immune response against them.

Raw milk also contains 22 amino acids, including eight that are considered essential. This means our body relies on foods to obtain them because it cannot produce them on its own. Additionally, our bodies cannot store amino acids, meaning that it needs a continuous supply. If even one amino acid is missing or damaged, the rest cannot function properly.

Kurt Oster, Chief of Cardiology and Chairman of the Department of Medicine at Park City Hospital in Bridgeport, CT states, "Milk has been changed over the years by processing into an unrecognizable, physiochemical emulsion, which bears very little resemblance to original, natural, and nutritional milk."

Why is milk pasteurized if it doesn't benefit those who drink it? Pasteurization turns a living food into a dead one and enables the milk to sit on store shelves for months. I have seen milk in stores dated six months from the expiration. In the case of ultra-pasteurization, refrigeration isn't needed until it is opened. Basically, putting it in the refrigeration section is for show. Consumers would likely have an issue looking for their milk and creamer next to the potato chips. This extended shelf-life benefits the producers and suppliers of the milk, not the health of the consumer. If you switch to fresh raw milk from cows raised outside on green grass, you will benefit yourself, the cow, and the farmer who sold it to you.

Mark McAffee of Organic Pastures, a raw milk dairy, has sold thousands of gallons of milk with no ill effects reported. Independent tests were performed between McAffee's raw milk and commercial pasteurized milk. Disease pathogens, including salmonella, listeria, and E.coli, were added to both the raw and the pasteurized milk. The raw milk, which contains beneficial bacteria, would not support the growth of pathogens and they all died off. However, in the pasteurized milk, the pathogenic bacteria thrived and proliferated. In the absence of the beneficial bacteria, harmful bacteria can more easily take hold.

Adding raw milk to your food regime will be essential for healing your digestive tract and eventually your disease. Raw organic pastured goat's milk is equally as beneficial as cow's milk. For additional information on raw milk, you can visit www.realmilk.com. This is also a great site to find raw milk producers in your area.

Raw Cheese
One of the best foods you can eat to bring more enzymes, vitamin B12, and good bacteria into your diet is cheese made from organic unpasteurized milk. In order for the cheese to contain vitamin B12, the cows that produced the milk must have been raised on pasture. This is because vitamin B12 is found in soil.

It is also important to pay attention to what your cheese is wrapped in. You may make the effort to buy organic raw cheese, but then find it is wrapped in plastic. Consumer's Union scientists found that out of 19 cheddar cheese samples, the seven packed in clear polyvinyl chloride (PVC) plastic cling wrap, such as Reynold's®, Saran Wrap®, or Glad Cling Wrap®, contained the plasticizer DEHA at an average of 153 parts per million (ppm) (Groth, 1998). This far exceeds the 18 ppm limit on food migration set by the Commission of the European Communities for DEHA. DEHA has been linked to birth defects and liver cancer in lab animals. Most of the DEHA from the plastic wrap ended up in the cheese. In fact, plasticizer molecules can migrate from packaging into food until they are depleted. Migration begins immediately.

Frustrating, isn't it? I order my cheese from James Ranch (www.jamesranch.net). It is set in one of the most beautiful, pristine environments you can imagine. The cheese comes in wheels that are sealed in wax. I slice the cheese as needed and place in glass lidded containers in the fridge for easy snacking. If you team up with friends or family who are taking this wonderful journey with you, you can share a wheel of cheese and shipping expenses.

Kefir
Kefir, which means "feel good" in Turkish, is an ancient, cultured, enzyme-rich food that is filled with friendly bacteria. It is made from whole organic raw milk and it will help you in ways nothing else can. Kefir is an essential part of your recovery. Here are some of the reasons why.

Although homemade yogurt is a perfectly healthy food, it doesn't hold a candle to kefir. Both are cultured milk products, but they work differently. The digestive enzymes in yogurt help digest the yogurt and only the yogurt. Kefir comes with extra enzymes that attach themselves to the walls of your gastrointestinal tract. The yogurt's nutrient delivery is gone in 24 hours, while kefir's is indefinite. It will fill your digestive tract with living, beneficial bacteria and enzymes.

Kefir contains 30-35 major strains of friendly bacteria not commonly found in yogurt. It is a turbo-charged, antibiotic colon cleanser. Kefir also contains beneficial yeasts, such as Saccharomyces kefir, which dominate and eliminate pathogenic yeasts. The beneficial yeasts penetrate the mucosal lining, where unhealthy yeast and bacteria reside, and destroy them. The friendly Candida yeast in kefir will kill the Candida albicans yeast that causes the classic yeast infection.

The complete proteins in kefir are partially digested and therefore more easily utilized by the body. Kefir is also rich in vitamin B12. You will have an immediate source of B12 to begin to heal. I cannot stress enough how important this is. Also, since the proteins are already partially digested, this will lessen the load on what little enzymes you are starting with. Your immune system will recognize these proteins and stop the attack. There just isn't another food out there that can match kefir for your specific needs.

Kefir also contains an ample supply of phosphorous, which aids your body in utilizing the proteins you are now able to break down for cell growth and energy. It is an excellent source of biotin, a B vitamin, which aids the body's absorption of other B vitamins (including B12). Kefir has a particularly calming effect on the nervous system. It contains calcium and magnesium, both of which are beneficial for healthy nerves and restful sleep. It also contains tryptophan, a precursor to serotonin and melatonin, well-known for their relaxing properties.

What if you are lactose intolerant? The lactose in kefir has already been predigested by the beneficial bacteria in the kefir. Therefore, even people with milk sensitivities can usually drink it. This is nature's perfect food.

A man-made probiotic supplement in pill form has around 15 million bacteria. Yes, that sounds like a lot, but if you look at 500 ml. of kefir, you get up to *five trillion* beneficial bacteria! The most difficult part of making kefir will be locating a source for organic raw pastured milk. Store bought kefir is made from pasteurized milk and contains denatured proteins.

In addition to the raw milk, you will need kefir grains (look in the resources section for where to order). Kefir grains are colonies of microorganisms, mostly yeasts and bacteria, that are beneficial to the human digestive tract. They form small, irregular, whitish balls, that when immersed in a nourishing liquid (usually raw milk), digest the liquid through a fermentation process that results in 'kefir.'

Once you have kefir grains, you then add the grains to the milk. Leave the milk on your kitchen counter overnight and you will have kefir within 1-2 days. Kefir resembles unsweetened yogurt in consistency and taste. Most likely you have never heard of kefir before reading this. It's just another casualty of our processed-food dependent generation. It has been consumed for centuries by some of the healthiest cultures in the world. You will soon be quite an expert in kefir and you will notice immediate improvements in your health and energy. Here is the recipe below.

KEFIR RECIPE

- Fill a quart jar within an inch of the top with milk.
- Add about a tablespoon of kefir grains.
- Cover jar loosely with cheesecloth and leave at room temperature.
- Swirl it once or twice a day to agitate the grains.
- It will probably take 1-2 days for the milk to thicken. It should have approximately the same consistency as yogurt.

That's it, you're done! I think it is best served very cold. I even chill my glass. Add fruit and honey, just as if you are making a smoothie. Enjoy!

STRAWBERRY-BANANA SMOOTHIE

- Homemade kefir
- 1 cup of organic strawberries
- 1 organic banana
- Honey to taste (we use organic raw honey)
- 1 teaspoon organic vanilla extract
- Ice

Blend all the ingredients except for the kefir together. Add the kefir last to minimize the blending and denaturing of the proteins.

ORANGE-BANANA SMOOTHIE

- Homemade kefir
- 1 organic banana
- 1 organic orange or large tangerine
- Honey to taste (we use organic raw honey)
- 1 teaspoon organic vanilla extract (optional)
- Ice

Blend all the ingredients except for the kefir together. Add the kefir last to minimize the blending and denaturing of the proteins.

Any dairy products made from pasteurized milk, such as store bought yogurt and kefir, will cause an immune response, since the pasteurization process will have damaged the proteins in the milk. In addition, all the beneficial bacteria and vital enzymes will have been destroyed. Every one of the 60 living enzymes is needed to bind and transport a corresponding nutrient in the milk. For instance, the enzyme lactoferrin binds the iron in the milk. Iron is a heavy metal ion and if it is not properly bound, it can harm normal cells and tissues.

Store bought yogurt and kefir have denatured proteins, no enzymes, no vitamin B12, and just a few strains of bacteria added back to replace the multitudes that were destroyed. This will just create more of an imbalance. They are not short cuts, they are dead ends.

Wine

"Do not drink water any longer, but use a little wine for the sake of your stomach and your frequent cases of sickness." 1 Timothy 5:23

Sounds like medical advice to me. Since we will be using wine as medicine, we will want it to be as close as possible to the wine mentioned in 1st Timothy. This means the wine should be organic or biodynamic; in other words, without added sulfites, fungicides, or pesticides. Compared with conventional wine, organic red wines have been found to have up to 30% higher levels of polyphenols, such as reservatrol, and antioxidant activities. A growing body of research worldwide, on the benefits of wine, has prompted the World Health Organization (WHO), the US government, and the American Heart Association to issue statements highlighting scientific findings associating health benefits with the moderate use of wine. The fermentation process of turning grapes into wine gives us a powerful medicine from nature. Only a little wine is recommended, and that is all that is needed.

Apple Cider

You likely have never had apple cider made the traditional way, even though it was at one time the most popular beverage in the country and certainly one of the healthiest. In the late 1700s, an average citizen consumed more than 35 gallons of cider annually. Every estate, farm, and property had a few apple trees or an apple orchard. That was usually one of the first things a homesteader did, plant his apple trees. John Adams attributed his health and long life to a tankard of cider before breakfast. "From the founding of Jamestown, to the time of George Washington and Thomas Jefferson, on down to that of Robert E. Lee, every plantation owner made cider, drank cider, and bragged about his cider," (Hedrick, 1988).

What passes for cider today is only a faint caricature of the cider our founding forefathers drank. Like raw cheese and milk, forced pasteurization has turned a truly healthful beverage into a sweet drink of little benefit to the human body. So why, in the past, was cider considered safer than water to drink? Because it was fermented.

I searched and searched in the United States, the land once so proud of its cider, and could find none that were prepared completely the traditional way. Some were organic and did ferment the apples for the proper time, but they did so in stainless steel tanks, not the wooden barrels that our forefathers used. The wooden barrels are what create some of the health benefits of the apple cider. The apples react with the wood to create enzymes. I did find an online source from France, *Organic Etienne Dupont*, for apple cider fermented in wood. The apples are from their own ancient orchard. I don't expect most of you to order in apple cider, but it is easy to make. Since there is a short list of truly fermented foods available, I thought I would include it. As demand increases, maybe we won't have to go to France to get our cider.

Apple Cider Vinegar

Apple cider vinegar is loaded with enzymes. If it agrees with you, then by all means, you should drink it. I would start with a little and work up; sip on it slowly. The apple cider you choose should be raw and organic. Bragg is a good brand. Just add ½ teaspoon of vinegar to a cup of warm, not hot, water.

Sauerkraut

Raw, organic, fermented sauerkraut will be vital to your recovery. Sauerkraut is thinly sliced cabbage which has been fermented. Its distinct sour flavor is the result of lacto-fermentation. Lactic acid, instead of vinegar, forms when bacteria in the fresh cabbage ferment the sugars. The art of preserving vegetables through fermentation goes back as far as 221 B.C., when it was discovered by the Chinese. Variants of fermented cabbage are used as food around the world.

Since neither refrigeration nor pasteurization is needed, the preservation of vegetables in this manner has provided man with a crucial source of nutrients in the winter for centuries. In fact, if the sauerkraut is pasteurized, all of the beneficial enzymes and lactic acid bacteria will be destroyed.

A healthy gut is very acidic and is populated with large numbers of beneficial bacteria. These bountiful, beneficial bacteria feed on the waste that remains from our digestion and create lactic acid. Our bodies depend on the lactic acid they produce to keep our gut healthy and in an acidic state. Without them, we would not have enough acidity to stop the growth of pathogenic parasites and yeasts. This can lead to an overgrowth of unfriendly yeasts, such as Candida albicans. Some of the symptoms of candida yeast overgrowth are fatigue, intense food cravings, gas, poor memory, bad breath, and indigestion. Lactobacilli plantarum is one of the beneficial strains of bacteria. It is found in only a few foods, but is abundant in sauerkraut. Lactobacilli plantarum is a dominant strain of probiotic bacteria that is known to actively aid in the digestive process. These strains of helpful bacteria also actively neutralize anti-nutrients, including phytic acid, which is found in all grains.

The same beneficial bacteria that create lactic acid in the gut are naturally present in cabbage. They are what is responsible for turning raw cabbage into nutrient dense, highly digestible sauerkraut. The process of fermentation dramatically increases the number of these microorganisms as they digest the cabbage and produce lactic acid. When we ingest the sauerkraut, we replenish our gut with the beneficial bacteria that have been created. In addition, the lactic acid in the sauerkraut will enable the new bacteria to thrive, and in turn create more lactic acid in our guts.

The lactic acid in sauerkraut will also partially compensate for reduced hydrochloric acid in our stomachs. That is why it can have such a profound and immediate effect on digestive woes.

Raw sauerkraut is also a potent nutritional medicine. Due to its many anti-oxidant compounds, sauerkraut has strong anti-carcinogenic properties. The cancer fighting ability of raw sauerkraut was recently confirmed by the results from a recent nutritional study conducted at the MTT Agrifood Research in Finland. The researchers made special note of the abundance of anti-oxidants, which are free radical scavengers useful in offsetting cellular damage that can lead to cancer. During the fermentation process, another nutrient, glucosinolate, is broken down by enzymes into powerful cancer-fighting compounds called isothiocyanates. In addition, sauerkraut contains large amounts of certain antioxidants like lutein and zeaxanthin; both are associated with preserving ocular health. Sauerkraut is also known to have antibacterial and antiviral properties. Sauerkraut also contains many vital nutrients and essential minerals. Among them are calcium, potassium, and magnesium. Vitamin C is also found in abundance.

Perhaps most important of all for the autoimmune sufferer, unpasteurized sauerkraut is very high in viable enzymes that work just like the ones from the pancreas. In fact, the bacteria in sauerkraut (Lactobacillus plantarum) have been analyzed by DNA fingerprinting and shown to produce nuclease (DNase I is a nuclease) and protease (Plengvidhya, 2007). For this reason, you should eat a little sauerkraut every time you consume protein. In general, all fermented foods can be said to aid in the assimilation and digestion of proteins, but perhaps none better than raw sauerkraut. This will be your medicine, so it should not be mass produced and it needs to be organic (Bubbie's® is not organic).

The fermented foods we are encouraging you to eat are just the beginning. There is a whole new world out there waiting for you to explore. Maybe you could plant some pickling cucumbers this summer and turn them into pickles for the winter. They could not be simpler to make and would be a wonderful addition to your new 'old world' way of eating. Food just doesn't get more nutritious than raw fermented foods. Every time you take a bite of this extraordinary medicine, you will be grateful that nature provided it for you to heal and to stay disease free.

We would like to share with you our own sauerkraut recipe. This recipe took us over a year to perfect. Enjoy!

GARLIC LEMON DILL SAUERKRAUT

Recipe courtesy of Christine Sanders and Kristin Urdiales

Ratios are based on a 7.5L crock. We use Harsch earthenware pickling crocks with a water reservoir. Harsch also makes a 5L crock. Many commercial sauerkraut purveyors have moved away from these old fashioned crocks and now use stainless steel or plastic. We believe, however, that these crocks are one of the reasons our sauerkraut is the best we have ever tasted.

To prepare your crock, first wash with a natural dish soap and then rinse thoroughly. You do not want to use anything strong or harsh, as the crocks can take on the taste and odor. Also wash the crock weights in the dishwasher and then soak them in white vinegar. This method has prevented any mold or yeast formation in our sauerkraut.

Ingredient List:

- 1 large bunch of fresh organic dill. You may need to preorder at your health food store.
- 1 large head of organic garlic
- 1 6.67 oz bottle of Volcano® brand organic lemon juice
- 10-11 lbs of organic green cabbage depending on the quality of cabbage. If the cabbage has a large core or is not tightly packed (has large air pockets), then less of it is usable and you will need closer to 11 lbs.
- 3-4 outer leaves of the cabbage
- sea salt

Preparing your ingredients for mixing:

Wash the cabbage thoroughly. Peel off the outer leaves of the cabbage and reserve to place on top of the cabbage at the end of the process. Halve the cabbage and take out the core. Cut the cabbage into the thickness of a dime.

Wash dill, cut up, place in a bowl and set aside. Mince garlic and mix with dill so that the garlic and dill are mixed evenly.

Put one pound of cut cabbage in a bowl with 1 heaping teaspoon of sea salt. Using your hands, or a potato masher, work the sea salt into the cabbage to release the cell sap. Continue kneading until moist, but do not overwork. Overworking will make the cabbage become limp and mushy.

Place the cabbage/garlic/dill mix into bottom of crock. Repeat the above process in one pound increments, layering the cabbage/garlic/dill in the crock as you go.

When you have finished the layering process and reached the top, wipe down any excess cabbage from the sides and the top of the crock to prevent mold.

Pour lemon juice over the top of the cabbage in the crock.

Now layer the outer leaves on top of the cabbage, so that none of it is exposed.

Place the crock weights on top of the cabbage and press down until the liquid rises above the stones. If the cabbage does not have a high enough moisture content to make the liquid rise above the stones, you will need to add a salt-water solution (33oz of water to 2 tbsp of sea salt mixed until salt is dissolved). Again wipe down any excess debris from the sides.

Put the lid on the crock and fill up the water well only half way. This water creates an air-tight barrier to prevent any dust, critters, etc. from getting into the sauerkraut. You will also know that it is fermenting by the air bubbles that begin rising in the water.

Place the crock on two boards, or use something to elevate it, so that air can circulate under the crock. For the first 3 days, place the crock in an area of your home that is approximately 68-72 degrees. After three days, the temperature is less critical, but at that temperature it will take approximately three weeks to become sauerkraut. At cooler temperatures, the process may take three and a half to four weeks. Look and listen for the air bubbles to know that it has begun fermenting.

You will periodically need to fill up the water well. Take care not to fill it so full that it gets into your sauerkraut.

After approximately three weeks, remove the lid, weights, and outer cabbage leaves carefully, so as not to contaminate the sauerkraut underneath. Place into jars and refrigerate. If the jars are unopened, the sauerkraut will last for 3-6 months. Once you begin opening the jar, it will last a week or two.

RAW FERMENTED SWEET PICKLE RELISH

We love this recipe because it is delicious and a great way to get another fermented food in your diet without any special equipment.

Ingredients:

- 1 cucumber
- ½ small red bell pepper (we use green bell peppers too)
- ½ teaspoon salt

Preparation:

Shred the veggies with a grater, food processor, or dice them finely. Put them in a jar with ½ teaspoon salt. Cap loosely or cover with cheesecloth and a rubber band and store in a cool dry place for three days or more. The warmer the storage place, the shorter the fermenting time. The texture should be crisp and the taste should be salty, sweet, and tangy. Replace the lid and refrigerate in between uses.

*This recipe came from www.goneraw.com

BEET KVASS

A sweet and salty lacto-fermented beverage infused with all of the vitamins, minerals, and detoxifying properties of beets.

Ingredients

- 5 large organic beets (any variety).
- 2 tbsp sea salt finely ground.

Preparation

1. Peel the beets. Chop them into one-inch cubes

2. Combine the sea salt and the chopped beets and place the mixture in a half-gallon jar.

3. Add enough water to fill the jar (well, spring, or filtered water is best), leaving about two-inches of space at the top. Stir to dissolve the salt and cover with a cloth or paper towel secured by a rubber band.

4. Allow to ferment in a warm spot of your kitchen for about 2 days before removing it to the refrigerator.

Nuts and Seeds

Nuts and seeds are a precious source of nutrition. They are brimming with enzymes. However, there is a caveat, you need to *soak* them. I know, that sounded strange to me too at first. Nuts and seeds naturally contain large amounts of enzyme inhibitors to keep them from sprouting before their appointed time. So, if you mistakenly drop a seed on your couch, it doesn't start growing. However, when you plant and water the seed, it does grow.

In nature, the growth cycle is triggered by rain. Nuts and seeds are waiting for this signal. The rain washes off the enzyme inhibitors, so it can germinate and grow into a plant. Soaking the nuts and seeds mimics this natural signal and washes away the enzyme inhibitors. This allows your body to benefit from all the vitamins and enzymes within the nuts and seeds. Nuts and seeds that are not soaked are very difficult to digest and will actually deplete your body's store of existing enzymes.

Soaking nuts and seeds was done by the people who came before us. It is the traditional method of preparation. The Aztecs would soak pumpkin and squash seeds in salt water and then dry them in the sun. This is still done today in parts of Central America. Since we are trying to restore enzymes and want to benefit from the wonderful store of nutrients and enzymes that nuts have to offer, we will want to soak them too.

NUT RECIPE BY SALLY FALLON

- 4 cups almonds (insecticide free is best)
- 1 tablespoon sea salt
- Filtered Water

Mix almonds with salt and cover with filtered water. Leave in a warm place for at least 7 hours or overnight. Drain in a colander. Spread on a stainless steel baking pan and place in a warm oven for around 24 hours (no more than 150 °F or 65 °C as this will kill the enzymes). Stir occasionally, until completely dry and crisp. Store in an air-tight container.

Skinless almonds will still sprout, indicating that the process of removing their skins has not destroyed the enzymes. Skinless almonds are easier to digest and more satisfactory in many recipes. However, you may also use almonds with skins on. You can use slivered almond pieces for this recipe.

You can also crisp peanuts, pine nuts, hazelnuts, macadamia nuts, cashews (as the enzymes in cashews are destroyed when they are processed it is best to roast quickly and soak no more than 6 hours). Makes 4 cups.

Raw Honey

Raw, organic honey should become your new sweetener. You can use it on your oatmeal in the morning, in your kefir smoothies, and for virtually anything else on which you would use sugar. Making sure it is raw and organic is vital, because not all honey is created equal.

Many chemicals can be used in producing non-organic honey. In addition, some honey producers are either feeding their bees corn syrup or adding corn syrup to the honey to increase profits. So, raw, organic honey is the only honey that we should be eating.

"Raw" means that it has not been heated to the point where all the beneficial enzymes have been killed. Raw, organic honey contains many health benefits. It helps with seasonal allergies, is antibacterial, boosts the immune system, and combats yeast overgrowth in the body.

In people with autoimmune disease that suffer with decreased amounts of pancreatic enzymes, the predigested sugar in honey is wonderful. The website www.honey-health.com describes how this predigestion is accomplished, "The consummation of this predigestive act is accomplished by the enzymes invertase, amylase, and catalase, which are produced by the worker bee in such large quantities that they can be found in every part of their bodies. However, there is plenty of it left in the honey for our benefit." We have provided a great source for raw honey in the resource section of this book, but you can also find wonderful local raw honey by visiting farmers' markets and using sources such as www.localharvest.org.

Give Up the Sugar, But Not the Chocolate!

The antioxidant benefits of dark chocolate have long been known, but now it is believed that raw cocoa directly feeds the beneficial bacteria in your GI tract. In addition to increased levels of beneficial bacteria, a preliminary clinical trial also observed an accompanying decrease in bacteria associated with diarrhea and constipation. Raw cocoa also decreased blood levels of triglycerides, cholesterol, and C-Reactive protein (a marker of inflammation associated with heart disease).

Cacao beans go through a fermentation process, so this might help explain their positive effect on bacterial levels in our guts. If you make your hot chocolate with enzyme rich honey, gut boosting cocoa powder, and raw milk, you will have a truly enjoyable way of replenishing your GI tract.

HONEY HOT CHOCOLATE

- 1 tablespoon raw honey
- 1 tablespoon organic raw cocoa
- 1 cup of raw milk

Mix together honey and cocoa into a paste. Add paste to the milk and heat slowly and gently on the stove until just hot. Do not allow to boil, as we want to keep as many beneficial bacteria and enzymes as we can. Add more honey and cocoa to taste. You can also make delicious chocolate milk with this recipe.

Instead of sugary juices and sodas, these are wonderful recipes for kids (and adults too).

LEMONADE RECIPE

- ½ cup raw honey
- ½ cup fresh squeezed lemon juice from organic lemons
- 1 cup water
- 4-6 cups more water to taste

Heat the ½ cup of honey and 1 cup of water together on stove until just dissolved. You want to heat as little as possible because heating the honey can kill beneficial enzymes. Then add lemon juice and the rest of the water to taste.

HOMEMADE POP

We modified this recipe from one we found on www.learningherbs.com. It has all of the taste and refreshment of our favorite fizzy drinks with none of the sugar or other additives. This lacto-fermented beverage is one of the most enjoyable ways to take in a fermented food. It is actually good for you!

Starter

- Add 1 tablespoon fresh grated ginger and 2 teaspoons raw honey to 1 quart cold water. Stir together. Cover with cheesecloth or an unbleached paper towel and secure with metal lid ring or a rubber band.
- Place on a cool part of the counter.
- Every day add 2 teaspoons of ginger and 2 teaspoons of honey and stir.
- After one week, cover with an air-tight lid. Place in the refrigerator.

Pop

Ingredients:

- 6 cups of fruit (strawberries, blueberries, rhubarb, etc. depending on what you want the flavor of the pop to be)
- 1 cup of raw organic honey
- 2 quarts cold water
- 1 cup of pop starter (see above)

Add fruit, honey, and cold water to pan. Warm just enough to dissolve the honey. Once honey is dissolved, allow mixture to cool and pour into a gallon jar and add 1 cup of pop starter.

*Do not add starter if mixture is too hot, as this will kill the live bacteria. Let cool until lukewarm.

Cover jar with cheesecloth or an unbleached paper towel. Let sit on the counter overnight. Strain into a clean jar and cover with an airtight lid. Refrigerate and enjoy!

Bone Broth and Clam Chowder

Science has confirmed what Grandma always knew, that broth made from bones is not just soup, but medicine. Bone broth is very soothing and healing to the GI tract. One of its main constituents is gelatin. Gelatin is a lubricating substance that lines the mucous membranes of the GI tract and guards against further damage.

Bone broth, used throughout history, has been affectionately called "Jewish Penicillin." It contains highly absorbable forms of calcium, magnesium, potassium, phosphorous, and sulfur, as well as trace minerals. Since it is soothing and highly nutritious, it will help restore your gut to health.

Store bought, canned soup will not do. You will need to make it the way Grandma did. You can simmer a big batch and freeze it for many meals to come. It really is not difficult or time consuming to make. I took some out of my freezer for dinner tonight. My favorite bone broth is chicken and rice. Here is the recipe:

CHICKEN AND RICE SOUP

- 1 whole chicken
- 2 celery ribs
- 2 cups cooked brown rice
- 2 large carrots
- 1 quartered onion
- 1 bay leaf

Wash the chicken well and put it in a large stock pot. Cover with water. Chop the carrots and celery into large chunks, quarter the onion and add to stock pot. Season with salt, pepper, and a bay leaf. Simmer for 2 hours or until chicken is tender.

Remove carrots, celery, and onion. Chop up the carrots into small chunks and add back to soup. Remove chicken, shred or dice, and add back to soup. Add 2 cups of cooked brown rice. That's it, you're done!

If you have a profound deficiency in vitamin B12, then you will need to eat proteins, at least temporarily, that contain very high levels of B12. The recommended dietary allowance (RDA) for vitamin B12 is 2.4 mcg. One chicken breast, one egg, and a cup of yogurt, for example, would need to be consumed daily just to meet the day's minimum requirement. There would be nothing left to make up the deficit that led to many of the symptoms associated with autoimmune disease.

Clams, oysters, and mussels all contain very high levels of B12. Clams provide the most with 98.9 mcg per 100 g serving. For a 3 oz serving, that would be 1401% of the RDA. Just one small clam would give you 156.6% of the RDA. If you make a big pot of clam chowder and freeze it in small shot-glass size containers, you could have an appetizer serving daily that would boost your B12 levels immensely. Just make sure to source your clams carefully. Sorry, canned clams won't do, as they contain high levels of bisphenol-A (BPA), a known endocrine disruptor that has been linked to cardiovascular disease, diabetes, obesity, and liver abnormalities. BPA is used to make polycarbonate plastic bottles and epoxy can linings. We have all heard about the dangers of plastic bottles, but a new study by researchers at Harvard School of Public Health found that people who ate just 12 ounces of canned soup for only 5 days had a 1,221% greater concentration of BPA in their urine (Carwile, 2011). The study's lead author stated that, "This study suggests that canned foods may be an even greater concern (than plastic bottles), especially given their wider use."

Next on the list would be organic pastured liver. The liver of almost any animal is loaded with B12 (B12 is stored in the liver). Lamb, beef, duck, and goose liver are all good choices. Lamb liver provides 72.85 mcg (230% RDA) in a 3 oz serving.

Caviar, octopus, fish, crab, and lobster all contain high amounts of B12, but are not in the same category as shellfish and liver. The proteins that most of us consume, such as beef, chicken, cheese, and eggs do have B12, and we will benefit by eating them, but an egg, for instance, has just 0.33 mcg per yolk or only 6% of the RDA.

No matter what protein you choose, the most important thing to remember is to consume it with a fermented vegetable, such as sauerkraut. Here is a recipe for my favorite clam (or oyster) chowder. Make a big pot and freeze some for many meals to come.

CLAM CHOWDER RECIPE

Ingredients:

1 quart shucked clams

1/3 pound salt pork

1 large white or yellow onion, minced

2 celery stalks, minced

2 large baking potatoes, diced

1 bay leaf

½ teaspoon thyme

1 quart half and half

½ cup unsalted butter (pastured raw butter is best), melted

¼ cup all-purpose flour

Coarse sea-salt

Fresh ground white or black pepper

Preparation:

- Drain and chop clams, reserving liquid.
- In a heavy pan, fry the salt pork until all fat is rendered.
- Toss in the onions and celery and brown lightly.
- Add the butter and flour and stir constantly for 5 minutes.
- Add potatoes, clam liquid, bay leaf, and thyme.
- Simmer the soup until potatoes are fork tender.
- Add chopped clams and half & half.
- Simmer 3-5 minutes.
- Allow to cool and freeze in glass containers.

*This recipe comes from www.clamchowderrecipe.net

The Green Smoothie

I wish I could take credit for this, but I can't. The credit for this delicious green drink, prepared in minutes, goes to Victoria Boutenko. She, like many of us, started to have health issues and knew she needed to change her way of eating. She also wanted and needed something that she actually enjoyed in order to keep doing it. Voila! The Green Smoothie was born. I know what you're thinking. Gross! Trust me, it's delicious. You can go to her website to hear her story and get some great recipes. I don't know her, and have never spoken to her, so her inclusion in this book will come as a surprise, I am sure.

Here is what is different about this vital green drink. It tastes good, and it combines only fruits and leafy greens. I have always avoided things that just didn't make sense. It didn't make sense to me to mix a whole bunch of things together in a blender that I wouldn't eat together at a meal. The starches in vegetables and the sugars in fruit don't combine well, at a meal, or in a blender. I would feel bloated and unwell if I ate the two together. Leafy greens don't contain starches and the fruit is not overpowered by them. The end result is that you taste all the sweetness of the fruit.

What I will take credit for is my personal green smoothie. Here is the recipe.

ANNESSE'S GREEN SMOOTHIE

- 2 slices of fresh ginger root (loaded with enzymes and anti-inflammatory properties)
- 1 kiwi (tons of enzymes)
- 1 tangerine
- 1 apple
- 1 handful baby spinach

Fill with water ¾ of the way up the blender. Blend and pour into a chilled glass. I drink this about four times a week.

You will find many more great recipes on Victoria's website www.rawfamily.com

We encourage you to eat a variety of organic fruits and vegetables. They will support the healing process and contribute many vital nutrients. Other healthy choices are organic beans, brown rice, quinoa, and lentils. The choices are endless. We like the cookbook *Nourishing Traditions* by Sally Fallon. It is filled with recipes for foods you were designed to eat. The important thing is to put careful thought and planning into the foods you feed yourself and your family.

Your Future

I promise, you have never had food like this. Your body most likely has never been truly nourished. Growing up, a typical school day lunch for me was a bologna sandwich on white bread and a Twinkie®. So, I know how foreign this new diet must sound. But when you start to eat living foods, your body will come alive too. It will also simplify your life. These foods are so satisfying, on such a deep level, that you won't crave processed food. Your brain won't constantly be sensing that it hasn't been nourished, and subsequently, keep driving you to eat more in order to find real nutrition. You will lose weight, you will lower your cholesterol, your blood sugars will normalize, your blood pressure will go down, and your energy will go up.

Nature gave us sauerkraut for winter, since we wouldn't have the fruit from fall trees or carrots from the summer gardens. Nature gave us cucumbers in the summer to be turned into pickles for the winter, so we would always have vital bacteria and enzymes. These are special foods. Nature has set them aside. They are unique in every way. Nothing can replace them; nothing else will do.

QUESTIONS AND ANSWERS

Q. Why does my hair fall out?
A. A strand of hair is composed of mostly protein, which means your hair needs protein to grow. Hair follicles have two states, a growth phase and a dormant stage. All hairs begin life in the growth phase and then shift into the dormant stage. The dormant stage lasts for about 100-120 days. After this, the hair will fall out. Normally, about 90 percent of hairs are in the growth phase and 10 percent are in the dormant stage. Specific stressors can result in a dramatic shift in the number of hairs into the dormant stage. Since autoimmune sufferers are unable to break down proteins, they would lack sufficient protein to maintain a healthy hair cycle. On a normal scalp, there are about 120,000-150,000 strands of hair, and about 50 to 100 strands are shed each day. That amount is hardly noticed by most people. If an unusually large number of hairs enter the dormant stage at the same time though, hair loss can become quite noticeable.

Two other nutrients that are found lacking in autoimmune sufferers would also play a significant role in hair loss. They are iron and zinc. Both iron and zinc are found in high protein foods and are necessary for the production of the various proteins that make up a strand of hair. Iron is the single nutrient most highly associated with hair loss. Zinc is a close second.

Q. Why are their ridges on my nails?
A. B12 deficiency shows up in several ways on the fingernail. It can manifest in a reduction in the visibility of the lunula, the "moon" at the base of your nail. Ridges can also be a sign of low B12.

Q. Why do women suffer with autoimmune diseases more than men?
A. There are two possible reasons, besides childbirth, that should be considered. The first reason is that women have a higher cellular turnover rate than men, which would leave more debris to be cleared from the body. This would create more opportunity for the immune system and enzymatic system to become overwhelmed and depleted. The second possible reason is that there are gender differences in protein metabolism.

Q. Why are there red dots on my skin?

A. They are called petechiae. Petechiae are caused by hemorrhages of small capillaries under the skin, due to endothelial cell damage. One disorder linked to petechiae is thrombocytopenia. Thrombocytopenia is a condition in which the blood has a lower than normal number of blood cell components called platelets.

In the research article entitled "Platelets, Petechiae, and Preservation of the Vascular Wall" it states that, "Platelets help to maintain blood circulation by controlling hemorrhage after an injury to the blood-vessel wall that causes physical or biochemical disruption of the endothelium," (Nachman, 2008). As we discovered in the section on homocysteine, homocysteine causes endothelial cells (the cells that line the inside of blood vessels, or endothelium) to commit "mass suicide".

Q. Why am I alcohol intolerant?

A. The enzyme responsible for the detoxification of alcohol is called alcohol dehydrogenase. Even under normal conditions, women make about 25% less of alcohol dehydrogenase than men. Alcohol dehydrogenase uses two molecular "tools" to perform its function, one of which is zinc. According to the National Institutes of Health Office for Dietary Supplements, the main source for zinc is animal–based protein foods, such as poultry, red meat, oysters, eggs, seafood, and milk (National Institutes of Health, 2010). The following studies confirm that autoimmune sufferers lack zinc:

1. Maes, M., I. Mihaylova, M. De Ruyter. 2006. Lower serum zinc in Chronic Fatigue Syndrome (CFS): relationships to immune dysfunctions and relevance for the oxidative stress status in CFS. J Affect Disorders 90(2-3):141-7.

2. Yilmaz, A., R.A. Sari, M. Gundogdu, N. Kose, E. Dag. 2005. Trace elements and some extracellular antioxidant proteins levels in serum of patients with systemic lupus erythematosus. *Clin Rheumatol* 24(4):331-5.

3. Palm, R., G. Hallmans. 1982. Zinc and copper in multiple sclerosis. J Neurol Neurosurg Psychiatry 45(8):691-8.

In the study "Dietary zinc-deficiency and its recovery responses in rat liver cytosolic alcohol dehydrogenase activities" it was concluded that, "These results suggest that rat liver cytosolic ADH activity was clearly related to dietary zinc intake levels," (Kawashima, 2011).

Q. What causes sleep apnea?

A. As far as the autoimmune disease process is concerned, sleep apnea has been linked to low dopamine and low acetylcholine. A study in Neurology found that patients with the lowest dopamine levels talked and thrashed while they slept (Gilman, 2003). Those with the lowest acetylcholine levels had the most interruptions in their breathing during sleep. This would make sense, acetylcholine controls the throat muscles.

Lack of acetylcholine could also lead to dysphagia. Dysphagia is difficulty swallowing, and along with sleep apnea, is a common condition in autoimmune disease.

Q: Why are there white spots on my skin?
A: This is called vitiligo. Patients with vitiligo develop white spots on the skin that vary in size and location. They are due to a lack of melanin. Melanin is a pigment that determines the color of skin, hair, and eyes. Melanin is produced in cells called melanocytes. If melanocytes cannot form melanin, skin color will become lighter or completely white as in vitiligo.

Melanin is synthesized in the body from the amino acid tyrosine. Tyrosine is derived from phenylalanine. Phenylalanine is an essential amino acid found in high protein foods. A lack of phenylalanine and tyrosine are commonly found in autoimmune sufferers, due to an inability to break down dietary proteins.

The skin's ability to tan also depends on an adequate supply of melanin. The body produces melanin in response to ultraviolet radiation and as a result tans the skin.

Q: Are allergies associated with autoimmune disease?
A: An allergic reaction is the body's way of dealing with an "invader." When the body senses a foreign substance, called an antigen, the immune system responds. The immune system normally protects the body from harmful agents such as bacteria and toxins. Its overreaction to a harmless substance, an allergen, is called a hypersensitivity reaction or an allergic reaction. When exposed to an allergen, B cells are alerted and turned into plasma cells, which produce Immunoglobulin E (IgE) antibodies to fight the invader. The IgE antibodies then attach themselves to mast cells via a receptor on the surface and remain attached. Upon subsequent exposure to the antigen, the mast cells release chemical mediators. The release of these chemical mediators from the mast cells is responsible for the allergic reaction.

IgE is an antibody that all of us have in small amounts. Allergic persons, however, produce IgE in large quantities. B12 stimulates TH1 suppressor T-cells, which then down regulate the overproduction of the allergen antibody IgE (Mansfield, Lyndon E. M.D. 1992). In addition, the chemical mediators released from the mast cells during an allergic response contain cytokines, such as tumor necrosis factor (TNF). The inability to modulate the chemical mediators, due to a lack of protease, would lead to a sustained and inappropriate response.

As stated earlier by Dr. Sarah Myhill, allergies to different foods can be triggered by poor digestion. If foods are poorly digested, large antigenically interesting molecules get into the lower gut and can initiate an immune response.

Q: How does the drug Plaquenil work?
A: Plaquenil works partly by blocking the activation of toll-like receptors on plasmacytoid dendritic cells. These cells produce antigens to DNA-containing immune complexes. These complexes result from the lack of DNase 1 to properly break down proteins and DNA, as we saw in the picture of the "lupus nets" in the beginning of the book.

Q: Why are lupus patients told to avoid alfalfa sprouts?

A: Alfalfa sprouts and seeds contain a protective chemical called canavanine. Just 0.2% canavanine can harm insect larvae. Canavanine is highly toxic to animals. Pigs will even refuse to eat feed containing too much canavanine.

"Canavanine interferes with the function of *enzymes and protein synthesis*," according to Dr. William Campbell Douglass. For this reason, canavanine has been linked in studies to the development of lupus-like symptoms in monkeys. In the abstract, "Systemic lupus erythematosus-like syndrome in monkeys fed alfalfa sprouts: role of a nonprotein amino acid," monkeys fed alfalfa seed developed a disease very similar to lupus. Additional research on this effect revealed that the monkeys recovered when the alfalfa seeds were no longer part of their diet. Additionally, there are published case reports of lupus patients suffering relapses after ingestion of alfalfa tablets. Alfalfa sprouts and seeds have a higher concentration of canavanine than the leaves or roots.

Q: Why do some drugs cause lupus?

A: Certain medications may cause lupus. This is called drug-induced lupus. There are 38 known medications that can cause drug-induced lupus. Most cases, however, are associated with procainamide (Pronesty), hydralazine (Apresoline), and quinidine (Quinaglute). All three of these drugs are *enzyme inhibitors*.

Q. Why does it seem as if a stressful event of some kind triggered your illness?

A. Both strenuous exercise and stress of any kind rapidly depletes your body of enzymes and B12. You could liken it to running a marathon. As you run, you become more and more exhausted, but you keep pushing yourself, and then you give an extreme push to reach the finish line, using up all of your reserves. If you are going through something stressful, you call on your already depleted body to produce even more. Then, as you cross the finish line, you collapse.

RESOURCES

Our resources are not 'big business', but rather small proprietors that are artisans of their craft. We know many of them personally and have spoken to them at length about how they make their products. We are sharing with you the things that are at our own dinner tables. Enjoy!

Sauerkraut, Pickles, and Other Vegetables

Kaptain's Kraut- Lemon Garlic Dill Sauerkraut and kefir grains- This is our favorite sauerkraut!
(425)443-7079

Happy Girl Kitchen Co.- canned tomatoes (in glass jars), classic dill pickles, and summer jam
www.HappyGirlKitchen.com/

Real Pickles- sauerkraut and pickles
www.RealPickles.com

Cultured Pickle Shop- sauerkraut
www.CulturedPickleShop.com
(510)540-5185

Thirty AcreFarm- sauerkraut, Kim chi, and real pickles
www.ThirtyAcreFarm.com

Milk, Kefir, and Cheese

Raw Milk- find resources in your area
www.RealMilk.com

Raw Cheese- organic, pastured cheese
www.JamesRanch.net

Kefir Grains- grains, jars and instructions
www.Etsy.com

Beef, Chicken, Pork and Shellfish

Good Earth Farms- organic, pastured beef, chicken, and pork
www.GoodEarthFarms.com

RESOURCES

Kachemak Shellfish Growers-for oysters grown in the pristine glacier-fed waters of Alaska   http://alaskaoyster.com/cm/

Dorsey Creek Organics-a wonderful family source for organic beef cattle, hogs, dairy cows, eggs, oats, spelt, rye, wheat, barley, corn, alfalfa seed, clover seed, and vegetable crops including rhubarb and asparagus.
http://www.dorseycreekorganics.com
stanjones53@hotmail.com or (307)-250-4325

Other Wonderful Finds

Living Nutz- organic germinated nuts
www.LivingNutz.com

Healing Spirits Herb Farm- one of the best herbalists in the country, and my mentor, Andrea Reisen   www.HealingSpiritsHerbFarm.com   (607)566-2701

Tropical Traditions- honey and organic coconut oil
www.TropicalTraditions.com

Northwest Wild Foods-wild blueberries, blackberries, huckleberries and more, perfect for your kefir smoothie or on your morning muesli.
http://www.nwwildfoods.com

Books and Resources

- **Nourishing Traditions** by Sally Fallon

- **Wild Fermentation** by Sandor Katz

- **The Raw Family** for more information on green smoothies and delicious recipes. www.RawFamily.com

- **Environmental Working Group** to find the toxicity rating of the beauty and bath products we use on our skin every day.
  http://www.ewg.org/skindeep/

- **Eat Wild** for information on where to find grass-fed foods in your area.
  www.EatWild.com

- **Local Harvest** is a great website to find many locally raised foods, including farmer's markets and CSA programs.
  www.LocalHarvest.org

REFERENCES

1. Abbott Laboratories. 2010. *What Causes Chron's Disease?* Humira. Retrieved 4/25/2011 from http://www.humira.com/crohns/causes.aspx

2. Addington, J.W. 1999. L-Serine: Treatment for Chronic Fatigue Syndrome (CFIDS). *ProHealth.* Retrieved 5/6/2011 from http://www.prohealth.com/library/showarticle.cfm?libid=428

3. Allen, R. 2004. Dopamine and iron in the pathophysiology of restless legs syndrome (RLS). *Sleep Med* 5(4):385-91.

4. Alsfasser G., B. Antoniu, S.P. Thayer, A.L. Warshaw, C. Fernández-del Castillo. 2005. Degradation and inactivation of plasma tumor necrosis factor-alpha by pancreatic proteases in experimental acute pancreatitis. *Pancreatology* 5(1):37-43.

5. Ambrosch, A., J. Dierkes, R. Lobmann, W. Kühne, W. König, C. Luley, H. Lehnert. 2001. Relation between homocysteinanemia and diabetic neuopathy in patients with Type 2 diabetes mellitus. *Diabet Med* 18(3):185-92

6. American Association for Cancer Research. 2005. *Broccoli Sprouts, Cabbage, Ginkgo Biloba and Garlic: A Grocery List for Cancer Prevention.* Retrieved 4/16/2011 from http://www.aacr.org/home/public--media/aacr-press-releases.aspx?d=553 (primary source). Source reference: Pathak, D.R. Joint association of high cabbage/sauerkraut intake at 12-13 years of age and adulthood with reduced breast cancer risk in polish migrant women: results from the US component of the Polish women's health study. Abstract number 3697. Presented at the AACR 4th Annual Conference on Frontiers in Cancer Prevention Research, October 30-November 2, 2005, Baltimore, Maryland.

7. American Diabetes Association. 2011. *Living with Diabetes: Autonomic Neuropathy.* Retrieved 6/01/2011 from http://www.diabetes.org/living-with-diabetes/complications/neuropathy/autonomic-neuropathy.html

8. American Heart Association. 1973. *Diet and Coronary Heart Disease.* American Heart Association. Dallas, TX.

9. Antonijević, N., M. Nesović, B. Trbojević, R. Milosević. 1999. Anemia in hypothyroidism. *Med Pregl* 52(3-5):136-40.

10. Aringer, M., J.S. Smolen. 2008. The role of tumor necrosis factor-alpha in systemic lupus erythematosus. *Arthritis Res Ther* 10(1):202.

11. Arthritis Today. 2009. *What is Fibromyalgia?* ArthritisToday.org. Retrieved 6/9/2011 from http://www.arthritistoday.org/conditions/fibromyalgia/all-about-fibro/what-is-fibromyalgia.php

12. Autoimmunity Research Foundation. 2009. Low Levels Of Vitamin D In Patients With Autoimmune Disease May Be Result, Not Cause, Of The Disease. *ScienceDaily.* Retrieved 4/3/2011 from http://www.sciencedaily.com /releases/2009/04/090408164415.htm

13. Aviña-Zubieta, J.A., H.K. Choi, M. Sadatsafavi, M. Etminan, J.M. Esdaile, D. Lacaille. 2008. Risk of cardiovascular mortality in patients with rheumatoid arthritis: A meta-analysis of observational studies. *Arthrit Care Res* 59(12):1690-7.

14. Avivi, I., N. Lanir, R. Hoffman, B. Brenner. 2002. Hyperhomocysteinemia is common in patients with antiphospholipid syndrome and may contribute to expression of major thrombotic events. *Blood Coagul Fibrin* 13(2):169-72.

15. Bakalar, N. 2008. Lack of vitamin B12 in elderly may cause brain shrinkage. The New York Times. Retrieved 03/03/2012 from http://www.nytimes.com/2008/09/09/health/09iht-09agin.16000758.html

16. Baltadzhieva, R., T. Gurevich, A.D. Korczyn. 2005. Autonomic Impairment in Amyotrophic Lateral Sclerosis. *Curr Opin Neurol* 18(5):487-93.

17. Baraniuk, J.N., B. Casado, H. Maibach, D.J. Clauw, L.K. Pannell, S. Hess. 2005. A chronic fatigue syndrome-related proteome in human cerebrospinal fluid. *BMC Neurol* 5:22.

18. Barba, A., B. Rosa, G. Angelini, A. Sapuppo, G. Brocco, L.A. Scuro, G. Cavallini. 1982. Pancreatic Exocrine Function in Rosacea. *Dermatology* 165:6.

19. Başkan, B.M., F. Sivas, L.A. Aktekin, Y.P. Doğan, K. Ozoran, H. Bodur. 2009. Serum Homocysteine Level in Patients with Ankylosing Spondylitis. *Rheumatol Int* 29(12):1435-9.

20. Bazzichi, L., L. Palego, G. Giannaccini, A. Rossi, F. De Feo, C. Giacomelli, L. Betti, L. Giusti, G. Mascia, S. Bombardieri, A. Lucacchini. 2009. Altered amino acid homeostasis in subjects affected by fibromyalgia. *Clin Biochem* 42(10-11):1064-70.

21. Beenakker, E.A., T.I. Oparina, A. Hartgring, A. Teelken, A.V. Arutjunyan, J. De Keyser. 2001. Cooling garment treatment in MS: clinical improvement and decrease in leukocyte NO production. *Neurology* 57(5):892-4

22. Beitzke, M., P. Pfister, J. Fortin, F. Skrabal. 2002. Autonomic dysfunction and hemodynamics in vitamin B12 deficiency. *Auton Neurosci* 18:97(1):45-54.

23. Benito-León, J., J. Porta-Etessam. 2000. Shaky-Leg Syndrome and Vitamin B12 Deficiency – case study. *New Eng J Med* 342(13):981.

24. Bennett, R. 2009. *Newly Diagnosed Patient*. National Fibromyalgia Association. Retrieved 6/9/2011 from http://www.fmaware.org/PageServer0bbc.html?pagename=fibromyalgia overview

25. Bernateck, M., M. Karst, K.F. Gratz, G.J. Meyer, M.J. Fischer, W.H. Knapp, W. Koppert, T. Brunkhorst. 2010. The First Scintigraphic Detection of Tumor Necrosis Factor-Alpha in Patients with Complex Regional Pain Syndrome Type I. *Anesth Analg* 110(1):2011-5.

26. Biagini, M.R., A. Tozzi, R. Marcucci, R. Paniccia, S. Fedi, S. Milani, A. Gali, E. Ceni, M. Capanni, R. Manta, R. Abbate, C. Surrenti. 2006. Hyperhomocysteinemia and Hypercoagulability In Primary Biliary Cirrhosis. *World J Gastroenterol* 12(10):1607-12.

27. Boras, W., J. Lukac, V. Brailo, P. Picek, D. Kordić, I.A. Zilić. 2006. Salivary interleukin-6 and tumor necrosis factor-alpha in patients with recurrent aphthous ulceration. *J Oral Pathol Med* 35(4):241-3.

28. Borland, S. 2011. Antibiotics increase risk of IBS and Chron's disease in children in later life. *The Daily Mail*, online. Retrieved 4/16/11 from http://www.dailymail.co.uk/health/article-1348044/Antibiotics-increase-risk-IBS-Crohns-disease-children.html

29. Bostom, A.G., I.H. Rosenberg, H. Silbershatz, P.F. Jaques, J. Selhub, R.B. D'Agostino, P.W. Wilson, P.A. Wolf. 1999. Nonfasting plasma total homocysteine levels and stroke incidence in elderly persons: the Framingham Study. *Ann Intern Med* 131(5):325-5.

30. Bowman, S.A., S.L. Gortmaker, C.B. Ebbeling, M.A. Pereira, D.S. Ludwig. 2004. Effects of fast-food consumption on energy intake and diet quality among children in a national household survey. *Pediatrics* 113(1): 112-18.

31. Broderick, K.E., V. Singh, S. Zhuang, A. Kambo, J.C. Chen, V.S. Sharma, R.B. Pilz, G.R. Boss. 2005. Nitric Oxide Scavenging by the Cobalamin (B12) Precursor Cobinamide. *J Biol Chem* 280(10):8678-85.

32. Caramaschi, P., N. Martinelli, D. Biasi, A. Carletto, G. Faccini, A. Volpe, M. Ferrari, C. Scambi, L.M. Bambara. 2003. Homocystein plasma concentration is related to severity of lung impairment in scleroderma. *J Rheumatol* 30(2):298-304.

33. Carbotte, R.M., S.D. Denburg, J.A. Denburg, C. Nahmias, E.S. Garnett. 1992. Fluctuating cognitive abnormalities and cerebral glucose metabolism in neuropsychiatric systemic lupus erythematosus. *J Neurol Neurosurg Psychiatry* 55(11):1054-9.

34. Carwile, J.L., X. Ye, X. Zhou, A.M. Calafat, K.B. Michels. 2011. *J Amer Med Assoc* 306(20):2218-20.

35. Catargi, B., F. Parrot-Roulaud, C. Cochet, D. Ducassou, P. Roger, A. Tabarin. 1999. Homocysteine, hypothyroidism, and effect of thyroid hormone replacement. *Thyroid* 9(12):1163-6.

36. Chajès, V., A.C.M. Thiébaut, M. Rotival, E. Gauthier, V. Maillard, M.C. Boutron-Ruault, V. Joulin, G.M. Lenoir, F. Clavel-Chapelon. 2008. Serum trans-monounsaturated fatty acids are associated with an increased risk of breast cancer in the E3N-EPIC Study. *Am J Epidemiol* 167(11):1312.

37. Chavarro, J.E., J.W. Rich-Edwards, B.A. Rosner, W.C. Willett. 2007. Dietary fatty acid intakes and the risk of ovulatory infertility. *Am J Clin Nutr* 85(1):231–7.

38. Chen, C.L., L.H. Tetri, B.A. Neuschwander-Tetri, S.S. Huang, J.S. Huang. 2011. A mechanism by which dietary trans fats cause atherosclerosis. *J Nutr Biochem* 22(7):649-55.

39. Chou, Y.C., M.S. Lee, M.H. Wu, H.L. Shih, T. Yang, C.P. Yu, J.C. Yu, C.A. Sun. 2007. Plasma homocysteine as a metabolic risk factor for breast cancer: findings from a case-control study in Taiwan. *Breast Cancer Res Tr* 101(2):199-205.

40. Cigna. 2010. *Vitamin B12*. Heathwise, Incorporated. Retrieved 6/5/2011 from http://www.cigna.com/healthinfo/hw43820.html

41. Clauw, D.J., M. Schmidt, D. Radulovic, A. Singer, P. Katz, J. Bresette. 1997. The relationship between fibromyalgia and interstitial cystitis. *J Pschiatr Res* 31(1):125-31.

42. Coates, T., J.P. Slavotinek, M. Rischmueller, D. Schultz, C. Anderson, M. Dellamelva, M.R. Sage, T.P. Gordon. 1999. Cerebral white matter lesions in primary Sjögren's syndrome: a controlled study. *J Rheumatol* 26(6):1301-5.

43. Constant, E.L., A.G. de Volder, A. Ivanoiu, A. Bol, D. Labar, A. Seghers, G. Cosnard, J. Melin, C. Daumerie. 2001. Cerebral Blood Flow and Glucose Metabolism in Hypothyroidism: A Positron Emission Tomography Study. *J Clin Endocrinol Metab* 86(8):3864-70.

44. Constantinescu, C.S. 2002. Migraine and Raynaud Phenomenon: Possible Late Complications of Kawasaki Disease. *Headache* 42(3):227-9.

45. Conti, F., V. Pittoni, P. Sacerdote, R. Priori, P.L. Meroni, G. Valesini. 1998. Decreased immunoreactive beta-endorphin in mononuclear leucocytes from patients with chronic fatigue syndrome. *Clin Exp Rheumatol* 16(6):729-32.

46. Cooke, J.P., D.W. Losordo. 2002. Nitric Oxide and Angiogenesis. *Circulation* (105):2133-5.

47. Dalakas, M.C., J. Hatazawa, R.A. Brooks, G. Di Chiro. 1987. Lowered cerebral glucose utilization in amyotrophic lateral sclerosis. *Ann Neurol* 22(5):580-6.

48. D'Ambrosi, A., A. Verzola, P. Buldrini, C. Vavalle, S. Panareo, S. Gatto, R. La Corte, L. Vicentini, A. Boccafogli, R. Scolozzi. 1998. Pancreatic duct antibodies and subclinical insufficiency of the exocrine pancreas in Sjögren's syndrome. *Recenti Prog Med* 89(10):504-9.

49. de Lau, L.M., A.D. Smith, H. Refsum, C. Johnston, M.M. Breteler. 2009. Plasma vitamin B12 status and cerebral white-matter lesions. *J Neurol Neurosurg Psychiatry* 80(2):149-57.

50. de Seze, J., T. Stojkovic, J.Y. Gauvrit, D. Devos, M. Ayachi, F. Cassim, T. Saint Michel, J.P. Pruvo, J.D. Guieu, P. Vermersch. 2001. Autonomic dysfunction in multiple sclerosis: cervical spinal cord atrophy correlates. *J Neurol* 248(4):297-303.

51. Dellwo, A. 2011. Dopamine in Fibromyalgia & Chronic Fatigue Syndrome. About.com. Retrieved 3/12/2012 from http://chronicfatigue.about.com/od/treatingfmscfs/a/dopamine.htm

52. Dewey, D.L. 1997. *The Facts About Canola Oil. Food For Thought.* Retrieved 6/7/2011 from http://www.dldewey.com/columns/canola.htm

53. Di Cagno, R., M. De Angelis, S. Auricchio, L. Greco, C. Clarke, M. De Vincenzi, C. Giovannini, M. D'Archivio, F. Landolfo, G. Parrilli, F. Minervini, E. Arendt, M. Gobbetti. 2004. Sourdough bread made from wheat and nontoxic flours and started with selected lactobacilli is tolerated in celiac sprue patients. *Appl Envirion Microbiol* 70(2):1088-96.

54. Dockser-Marcus, A. 2011. A step closer to tests for chronic fatigue syndrome and Lyme disease. *The Wall Street Journal: Health Blog.* Retrieved 4/25/2011 from http://blogs.wsj.com/health/2011/02/23/a-step-closer-to-tests-for-chronic-fatigue-syndrome-and-lyme-disease/

55. Donaldson, J.O., M.L. Grunnet, H.G. Thompson. 1983. Concurrence of Myasthenia Gravis, Thymoma, and Thyroid Carcinoma. *Arch Neurol* 40(2):122-4.

56. Dong, M., Y. Shi, Q. Cheng, M. Hao. 2001. Increased nitric oxide in peritoneal fluid from women with idiopathic infertility and endometriosis. *J Repro Med* 46(10):887-91.

57. Ebbing, M., K.H. Bønna, O. Nygård, E. Amesen, P.M. Ueland, J.E. Nordrehaug, K. Rasmussen, I. Njølstad, H. Refsum, D.W. Nilsen, A. Tverdal, K. Meyer, S.E. Vollset. 2009. Cancer incidence and mortality after treatment with folic acid and vitamin B12. *J Amer Med Assoc* 18;302(19):2119-26.

58. Edwards, Rob. 2002. Farm salmon is now most contaminated food on shelf; Nationwide. *Sunday Herald*, 20 October 2002. Retrieved 2-20-11 from http://www.robedwards.com/2002/10/farm_salmon_is_.html

59. Environmental Working Group. 2012. *Skin Deep Cosmetics Database.* EWG.org. Retrieved 3/14/2012 from http://www.ewg.org/skindeep/

60. Fallon, S. 2008. Puffed Grains and Breakfast Cereals, should we eat them? *Nourished Magazine – Editor's Blog.* Retrieved 2/21/2011 from http://editor.nourishedmagazine.com.au/articles/puffed-grains-should-we-eat-them

61. Fallon, S. 2003. *Nourishing Traditions: The Cookbook that Challenges Politically Correct Nutrition and the Diet Dictocrats.* Newtrends Publishing, Inc: Winona Lake, IN.

62. Fallon, S., M.G. Enig. 2005. Vitamin B12: Vital Nutrient for Good Health. Weston A. Price Foundation. Retrieved 5/9/2011 from www.westonaprice.org/viamins-and-minerals/vitamin-b12.

63. Finsen, B., J. Antel, T. Owens. 2002. TNFa: kill or cure for demylinating disease? *Mol Psychiatr* 7:820-1.

64. Food and nutrition board, institute of medicine of the national academies. 2005. *Dietary Reference Intakes for Energy, Carbohydrate, Fiber, Fat, Fatty Acids, Cholesterol, Protein, and Amino Acids (Macronutrients).* National Academies Press: Washington, D.C.

65. Franz, B., C. Anderson. 2007. The potential role of joint injury and eustachian tube dysfunction in the genesis of secondary Ménière's disease. *Int Tinnitus J* 13(2):132-7.

66. Fukumura, D., T. Gohongi, A. Kadambi, Y. Izumi, J. Ang, C.O. Yun, D.G. Buerk, P.L. Huang, R.K. Jain. 2001. Predominant role of endothelial nitric oxide synthase in vascular endothelial growth factor-induced angiogenesis and vascular permeability. *P Natl Acad Sci USA* 98(5):2604-9.

67. Gazquez, I., A. Aoro-Varela, I. Aran, S. Santos, A. Batuecas, G. Trinidad, H. Perez-Garrigues, C. Gonzalez-Oller, L. Acosta, J.A. Lopez-Escamez. 2011. High Prevalence of Systemic Autoimmune Diseases in Patients With Ménière's Disease. *PLoS One* 6(10):e26759.

68. Gerhard, G.T., P.B. Duell. 1999. Homocysteine and atherosclerosis. *Curr Opin Lipidol* 10(5):417-28.

69. Ghosh, S., S.N. Kabir, A. Pakrashi, S. Chatteriee, B. Chakravarty. 1993. Subclinical Hypothyroidism: A Determinant of Polycystic Ovary Syndrome. *Horm Res* 39(1-2):61-6.

70. Gilman, S., R.D. Chervin, R.A. Koeppe, F.B. Consens, R. Little, H. An, L. Junck, M. Heumann. 2003. Obstructive sleep apnea is related to a thalamic cholinergic deficit in MSA. *Neurology* 61(1):35-9.

71. Giovannoni, G., N.C. Silver, J. O'Riordan, R.F. Miller, S.J. Heales, J.M. Land, M. Elliot, M. Feldmann, D.H. Miller, E.J. Thompson. 1999. Increased urinary nitric oxide metabolites in patients with multiple sclerosis correlates with early and relapsing disease. *Mult Scler* 5(5):335-41.

72. Gleason, M.N., R.E. Gosselin, H.C. Hodge. 1957. *Clinical Toxicology of Commercial Products: Acute Poisoning, Home & Farm Edition.* The Williams & Wilkins Co.:Baltimore, M.D.

73. Gocer, C., U. Genc, A. Eryilmaz, A. Islam, S. Boynuegri, F. Bakir. 2009. Homocysteine, Folate and Vitamin B12 Concentrations in Middle Aged Adults Presenting With Sensorineural Hearing Impairment. *J Int Adv Otol* 5(3):340-4.

74. Gonzalez, F., K. Thusu, E. Abdel-Rahman, A. Prabhala, M. Tomani, P. Dandona. 1999. Elevated Serum Levels of Tumor Necrosis Factor Alpha in Women with Polycystic Ovary Syndrome. *Metabolism* 48(4):437-41.

75. González, R., T. Pedro, J.T. Real, S. Martínez-Hervás, M.R. Abellán, R. Lorente, A. Priego, M. Catalá, F.J. Chaves, J.F. Ascaso, R. Carmena. 2010. Plasma homocysteine levels are associated with ulceration of the foot in patients with type 2 diabetes mellitus. *Diabetes Metab Res Rev* 26(2):115-20.

76. Gorman, J.D., K.E. Sack, J.C. Davis. 2002. Treatment of Ankylosing Spondylitis by Inhibition of Tumor Necrosis Factor Alpha. *New Engl J Med* 346(18):1349-56.

77. Graham, D.N. 2008. *Nutrition and Athletic Performance*; 2nd edition. Food 'n' Sport Press:Marathon, FL.

78. Grant, R. 2002. Fermenting Sauerkraut Produces Stronger Cancer Fighter. *HealthScoutNew*s. Retrieved 6/7/2011 from http://www.rense.com/general30/fermentingsauerkraut.htm

79. Greco, L., M. Gobbetti, R. Auricchio, R. Di Mase, F. Landolfo, F. Paparo, R. Di Cagno, M. De Angelis, C.G. Rizzello, A. Cassone, G. Terrone, L. Timpone, M. D'Aniello, M. Maglio, R. Troncone, S. Auricchio. 2011. Safety for patients with celiac disease of baked goods made of wheat flour hydrolyzed during food processing. *Clin Gastroenterol Hepatol* 9(1):24-9.

80. Groth, E. III, 1998. *Report*. Consumers Union. Retrieved 4/3/11 from http://www.consumersunion.org/food/plasticny698.htm

81. Guengerich, F.P. 2008. Cytochrome p450 and chemical toxicology. *Chem Res Toxicol* 21(1):70-83.

82. Gunal, D.I., N. Afsar, T. Tanridag, S. Aktan. 2002. Autonomic dysfunction in multiple sclerosis: Correlation with disease-related parameters. *Eur Neurol* 48(1):1-5.

83. Hakkim, A., B.G. Fürnrohr, K. Amann, B. Laube, U.A. Abed, V. Brinkmann, M. Herrmann, R.E. Voll, A. Zychlinsky. 2010. Impairment of NET degradation is associated with Lupus nephritis. *P Natl Acad Sci* 107(21):9813-18.

84. Harel, Z., G.S. Tannenbaum. 1993. Dietary protein restriction impairs both spontaneous and growth hormone-releasing factor-stimulated growth hormone release in the rat. *Endocrinology* 133(3):1035-43.

85. Harvard School of Public Health. 2007. Higher Trans Fat Levels In Blood Associated With Elevated Risk Of Heart Disease. *ScienceDaily*. Retrieved April 3, 2011, from http://www.sciencedaily.com /releases/2007/03/070327144449.htm

86. Hassan, C., A. Zullo, V. De Francesco, S.M. Campo, S. Morini, C. Panella, E. Ierardi. 2007. Tumor necrosis factor alpha in ulcerative colitis and diverticular disease associated colitis. *Endocr Metab Immune Disord Drug Targets* 7(3):187-94.

87. Hattemer, P. 2002. *The Health Forum--Book 2: Canadidiasis and Dysbiosis: Albatement Techniques*. Health Reflections Book Corp: Manhattan Beach, CA. Retrieved 4/16/2011 from http://www.scribd.com/doc/3484586/Polly-Hattemer-Book-2-Ttreatments

88. He, L., H. Zeng, F. Li, J. Feng, S. Liu, J. Liu, J. Yu, J. Mao, T. Hong, A.F. Chen, X. Wang, G. Wang. 2010. Homocysteine impairs coronary artery endothelial function by inhibiting tetrahydrobiopterin in patients with hyperhomocysteinemia. *Am J Physiol Endocrinol Metab* 299(6):E1061-5.

89. Hedrick, U.P. 1988. A history of horticulture in America to 1860. Portland, Oregon: Timber Press.

90. Herrlinger, K.R., E.F. Stange. 2000. The pancreas and inflammatory bowel diseases. *Int J Pancreatol* 27(3):171-9.

91. Higdon, J. 2003. Coenzyme Q10. Linus Pauling Institute, Oregon State University. Retrieved 12/26/2011 from http://lpi.oregonstate.edu/infocenter/othernuts/coq10/

92. Hilker, R., A. Thiel, C. Geisen, J. Rudolf. 2000. Cerebral blood flow and glucose metabolism in multi infarct-dementia related to primary antiphospholipid antibody syndrome. *Lupus* 9(4):311-6.

93. Holman, R.T., S.B. Johnson, E. Kokmen. 1989. Deficiencies of polyunsaturated fatty acids and replacement by nonessential fatty acids in plasma lipids in multiple sclerosis. *P Natl Acad Sci USA* 86(12):4720-4.

94. Hooper, D.C., S. Spitsin, R.B. Kean, J.M. Champion, G.M. Dickson, I. Chaudhry, H. Koprowski. 1998. Uric acid, a natural scavenger of peroxynitrite, in experimental allergic encephalomyelitis and multiple sclerosis. *P Natl Acad Sci USA* 95(2):675-80.

95. Hooshmand, B., A. Solomon, I. Kåreholt, J. Leiviskä, M. Rusanen, S. Ahtiluoto, B. Winblad, T. Laatikainen, H. Soininen, M. Kivipelto. 2010. Homocysteine and holotranscobalamin and the risk of Alzheimer disease: a longitudinal study. *Neurology* 75(16):1408-14.

96. Hörl, W.H. 2008. New insights into intestinal iron absorption. *Nephrol Dial Transplant* 23(10):3063-4.

97. Houghton Mifflin. 2007. *The American Heritage Medical Dictionary*. Houghton Mifflin Company: Boston, MA. Retrieved 5/9/2011 from http://medical-dictionary.thefreedictionary.com/atherogenic

98. Hyman, M. 2009. Autoimmune Disease: How to stop your body from attacking itself. *Huffpost Living*. Retrieved 4/3/11 from http://www.huffingtonpost.com/dr-mark-hyman/autoimmune-disease-how-to_b_283707.html?page=4&show_comment_id=30909196

99. Iłżecka, J., Z. Stelmasiak, J. Solski, S. Wawrzycki, M. Szpetnar. 2003. Plasma amino acids percentages in amyotrophic lateral sclerosis patients. *Neurol Sci* 24(4):293-5.

100. Institute of Health Science. 2010. *80% of your Immune System is actually in your GI Tract*. Retrieved 4/3/2011 from http://www.instituteofhealthsciences.com/80-of-your-immune-system-is-actually-in-your-gi-tract/

101. Institute of Medicine/National Academies. 2010. Report sets new dietary intake levels for calcium and vitamin D to maintain health and avoid risks associated with excess. *ScienceDaily*. Retrieved 4/3/2011, from http://www.sciencedaily.com /releases/2010/12/101201152802.htm

102. International Scleroderma Network. 2011. *Overview of Scleroderma Dental Involvement*. Sclero.org. Retrieved 6/9/2011 from http://sclero.org/medical/symptoms/dental/a-to-z.html

103. Jabbar, A., A. Yawar, S. Waseem, N. Islam, N. Ul Haque, L. Zuberi, A. Khan, J. Akhter. 2009. Vitamin B12 deficiency common in primary hypothyroidism. *J Pak Med Assoc* 59(2):126.

104. Jason, L.A., K. Corradi, S. Gress, S. Williams, S. Torres-Harding. 2006. Causes of Death Among Patients with Chronic Fatigue Syndrome. *Health Care Women Int* 27:615-26.

105. Johns Hopkins Lupus Center. 2011. *Throid Medications*. Johns Hopkins Medicine. Retrieved 6/9/2011 from http://www.hopkinslupus.org/lupus-treatment/common-medications-conditions/thyroid-medications/

106. Johns Hopkins Lupus Center. 2012. Johns Hopkins Medicine, Internet. Retrieved 4/28/12 from http://www.hopkinslupus.org/lupus-info/lifestyle-additional-information/lupus-cancer/ Johnson, C. 2010. *Proteins on the Brain: Spinal Tapping for ME/CFS*. The Environmental Illness Resource. Retrieved 6/5/2011 from http://www.ei-resource.org/columns/phoenix-rising/proteins-on-the-brain:-spinal-tapping-for-cfs/

107. Jones, F.T. 2007. A Broad View of Arsenic. *Poultry Science* 86(1):2-14.

108. Jones, M., D.C. Kennedy. 1998. *Food and Beverage Sources of Fluoride Exposure*. NoFluoride.com. Retrieved 2/19/2011 from http://www.nofluoride.com/presentations/Fluoride_content_food_%26_beverages.pdf

109. Kamburoglu, G., K. Gumus, S. Kadayifcilar, B. Eldem. 2006. Plasma homocysteine, vitamin B12 and folate levels in age-related macular degeneration. *Graefes Arch Clin Exp Ophthalmol* 244(5):565-9.

110. Kang, A.H., R.L. Trelstad. 1973. A Collagen Defect in Homocystinuria. *J Clin Invest* 52(10):2571-8.

111. Kawashima, S., M. Yokoyama. 2004. Dysfunction of endothelial nitric oxide synthase and atherosclerosis. *Arterioscler Thromb Vasc Biol* 24(6):998-1005.

112. Kawashima, Y., Y. Someya, S. Sato, K. Shirato, M. Jinde, S. Ishida, S. Akimoto, K. Kobayashi, Y. Sakakibara, Y. Suzuki, K. Tachiyashiki, K. Imaizumi. Dietary zinc-deficiency and its recovery responses in rat liver cytosolic alcohol dehydrogenase activities. *J Toxicol Sci* 36(1):101-8.

113. Keay, S.K., Z. Szekely, T.P. Conrads, T.D. Veenstra, J.J. Barchi Jr, C.O. Zhang, K.R. Koch, C.J. Michejda. 2004. An antiproliferative factor from interstitial cystitis patients is a frizzled 8 protein-related sialoglycopeptide. *Proc Natl Acad Sci USA* 101(32):11803-8.

114. Kirschmann, D.A., K.L. Duffin, C.E. Smith, J.K. Welply, S.C. Howard, B.D. Schwartz, S.L. Woulfe. 1995. Naturally processed peptides from rheumatoid arthritis associated and non-associated HLA-DR alleles. *J Immunol* 155(12):5655-62.

115. Kocer, B., S. Engur, F. Ak, M. Yilmaz. 2009. Serum vitamin B12, folate, and homocysteine levels and their association with clinical and electrophysiological parameters in multiple sclerosis. *J Clin Neurosci* 16(3):399-403.

116. Koskela, L.R., N.P. Wiklund. 2007. Nitric Oxide in the Painful Bladder/Interstitial Cystitis. *J Urol Urogynäkol* 14(1):18-9.

117. Krauss, R.M., R.H. Eckel, B. Howard, L.J. Appel, S.R. Daniels, R.J. Deckelbaum, J.W. Erdman, P. Kris-Etherton, I.J. Goldberg, T.A. Kotchen, A.H. Lichtenstein, W.E. Mitch, R. Mullis, K. Robinson, J. Wylie-Rosett, S. St. Jeor, J. Suttie, D.L. Tribble, T.L. Bazzarre. 2000. AHA Dietarty Guidelines: Revision 2000: A Statement for healthcare professionals from the Nutrition Committee of the American Heart Association. *Circulation* 102:2284-99.

118. Kritchevsky, S.B. 2004. A Review of Scientific Research and Recommendations Regarding Eggs. *J Am Coll Nutr* 23(6):596S-600S.

119. Krishnaveni, G.V., J.C. Hill, S.R. Veena, D.S. Bhat, A.K. Wills, C.L. Karat, C.S. Yajnik, C.H. Fall. 2009. Low plasma vitamin B12 in pregnancy is associated with gestational 'diabesity' and later diabetes. *Diabetologia* 52 (11):2350-8.

120. Krueger, G., K. Callis. 2004. Potential of Tumor Necrosis Factor Inhibitors in Psoriasis and Psoriatic Arthritis. *Arch Dermatol* 140:218-25.

121. Lammers, K., S.L. Lince, M.A. Spath, L.C. van Kempen, J.C. Hendriks, M.E. Vierhout, K.B. Kluivers. 2012. Pelvic organ prolapse and collagen-associated disorders. *Int Urogynecol J* 23(3):313-9.

122. Latimer, E. 2009. Spraying for bugs could increase autoimmune disease risk - Press Release. *American College of Rheumatology*. Retrieved 2/19/11 from https://www.rheumatology.org/about/newsroom/2009/2009_am_18.asp

123. Lazzerini, P.E., P.L. Capecchi, S. Bisogno, M. Cozzalupi, P.C. Rossi, F.L. Pasini. 2010. Homocysteine and Raynaud's phenomenon: a review. *Autoimmun Rev* 9(3):181-7.

124. Lee, L. 2009. *Arthritis*. LitaLee.com Retrieved 2/19/11 from http://www.litalee.com/shopexd.asp?id=132

125. Leem, J., E.H. Koh. 2012. Interaction between mitochondria and the endoplasmic reticulum: implications for the pathogenesis of type 2 diabetes mellitus. *Exp Diabetes Res* 2012:242984.

126. Levy, Y., J. George, P. Langevitz, D. Harats, R. Doolman, B.A. Sela, Y. Shoenfield. 1999. Elevated homocysteine levels in patients with Raynaud's syndrome. *J Rheumatol* 26:2383-5.

127. Li, W., T. Zheng, J. Want, B.T. Altura, B.M. Altura. 1999. Extracellular magnesium regulates effects of vitamin B6, B12 and folate on homocysteinemia-induced depletion of intracellular free magnesium ions in canine cerebral vascular smooth muscle cells: possible relationship to [Ca2+]i, atherogenesis and stroke. *Neurosci Lett* 274(2):83-6.

128. Litwic, A., E. Dennison. 2010. *Osteoporosis in Rheumatoid Arthritis*. National Rheumatoid Arthritis Society. Retrieved 03/03.2012 from http://www.nras.org.uk/about_rheumatoid_arthritis/established_disease/possible_complications/osteoporosis_in_ra.aspx

129. Long, C., T. Alterman. 2007. Meet Real Free-Range Eggs. *Mother Earth News*. Retrieved 4/16/2011 from http://www.motherearthnews.com/Real-Food/2007-10-01/Tests-Reveal-Healthier-Eggs.aspx

130. Lopez-Garcia, E., M.B. Schulze, J.B. Meigs, J.E. Manson, N. Rifai, M.J. Stampfer, W.C. Willett, F. B. Hu. 2005. Consumption of Trans Fatty Acids Is Related to Plasma Biomarkers of Inflammation and Endothelial Dysfunction. *J Nutr* 135(3):562–6.

131. Lord, S.R., J.A. Bralley. 1994. Treatment of Chronic Fatigue Syndrome with Specific Amino Acid Supplementation. *J Appl Nutr* 46(3):74-8.

132. Lorenzo Gómez, M.F., S. Gómez Castro. 2004. [Physiopathologic relationship between interstitial cystitis and rheumatic, autoimmune, and chronic inflammatory diseases]. *Arch Esp Urol* 57(1):25-34.

133. Loverro, G., F. Lorusso, L. Mei, R. Depalo, G. Cormio, L. Selvaggi. 2002. The Plasma Homocysteine Levels are Increased in Polycystic Ovary Syndrome. *Gynecol Obstet Invest* 53(3):157-62

134. Lu, S.C., C.H. Shih, T.H. Liao. 2003. Expression of DNase I in Rat Parotid Gland and Small Intestine is Regulated by Starvation and Refeeding. *J Nutr* 133:71-4.

135. Lundström, I.M., F.D. Lindström. 2001. Iron and vitamin deficiencies, endocrine and immune status in patients with primary Sjögren's syndrome. *Oral Dis* 7(3):144-9.

136. Lupus Foundation of America. 2011. *Living With Lupus: Pain.* Lupus Foundation of America, Inc. Retrieved 6/9/2011 from http://www.lupus.org/webmodules/webarticlesnet/templates/new_learnliving.aspx?articleid=2255&zoneid=527

137. Machado, D.E., P.T. Berardo, C.Y. Palmero, L.E. Nasciutti. 2010. *J Exp Clin Canc Res* 29:4.

138. Maes, M., I Mihaylova, M. Kubera, M. Uytterhoeven, N. Vrydags, E. Bosmans. 2009. Coenzyme Q10 deficiency in myalgic encephalomyelitis/chronic fatigue syndrome (ME/CFS) is related to fatigue, autonomic and neurocognitive symptoms and is another risk factor explaining the early mortality in ME/CFS due to cardiovascular disorder. *Neuro Endocrinol Lett* 30(4):470-6.

139. Maes, M., I. Mihaylova, M. De Ruyter. 2006. Lower serum zinc in Chronic Fatigue Syndrome (CFS): relationships to immune dysfunctions and relevance for the oxidative stress status in CFS. *J Affect Disorders* 90(2-3):141-7.

140. Mahfouz, M. 1981. Effect of dietary trans fatty acids on the delta 5, delta 6 and delta 9 desaturases of rat liver microsomes in vivo. *Acta Biol Med Ger* 40(12):1699–1705.

141. Makino, T., H. Kawashima, H. Konishi, T. Nakatani, H. Kiyama. 2010. Elevated Urinary Levels and Urothelial Expression of Hepatocarcinoma-intestine-pancreas/Pancreatitis-associated Protein in Patients with Interstitial Cystitis. *Urology* 75(4):933-7.

142. Makris, A., H. Cladd, R.J. Burcombe, J.M. Smith, M. Makris, 2001. Raised Plasma Homocysteine Levels in Women with Metastatic Breast Cancer. *Proc Am Soc Clin Oncol* 20:Abstract 179.

143. Mandl, T., V. Granberg, J. Apelqvish, P. Wollmer, R. Manthrope, L.T.H. Jacobsson. 2008. Autonomic nervous symptoms in primary Sjögren's syndrome: a follow-up study. *Rheumatology* 47:914-9.

144. Mann, D.L., D.R. Siegfried. 2011. The Diabetes-Arthritis Connection. *Arthritis Today*. Retrieved 6/9/2011 from http://www.arthritistoday.org/conditions/more-conditions/diabetes-arthritis.php

145. Marcoullis G., Y. Parmentier, J.P. Nicolas, M. Jimenez, P. Gerard. 1980. Cobalamin Malabsorption Due to Nondegradation of R Proteins in the Human Intestine. *J Clin Invest* 66(3):430–40.

146. Martinez-Lavín, M. 2001. A Novel Holistic Explanation for the Fibromyalgia Enigma: Autonomic Nervous System Dysfunction. *Fibromyalgia Frontiers* 10(1).

147. Mayfrank, L., U. Thoden. 1986. Downbeat nystagmus indicates cerebellar or brain-stem lesions in vitamin B12 deficiency. *J Neurol* 233(3):145-8.

148. Mayo Clinic staff. 2009. *Raynaud's disease*. Mayo Clinic. Retrieved 6/9/2011 from http://www.mayoclinic.com/health/raynauds-disease/DS00433/DSECTION=causes

149. McBride, J. 2000. *B12 deficiency may be more widespread than thought*. USDA Agricultural Research Service. Retrieved 4/3/11 from http://www.ars.usda.gov/is/pr/2000/000802.htm

150. McCormick, J. 2005. A possible link between $24-billion-a-year "antacid" industry and the misery of menopause. *MSNBC News*. Retrieved 4/16/2011 from http://www.msnbc.msn.com/id/40423327/ns/health-diabetes/

151. McLean, R.R., P.F. Jacques, J. Selhub, K.L. Tucker, E.J. Samelson, K.E. Broe, M.T. Hannan, L.A. Cupples, D.P. Kiel. 2004. Homocysteine as a predictive factor for hip fracture in older persons. *New Engl J Med* 350(20):2042-9.

152. Merck & Co., Inc. 2011. *The Merck Veterinary Manual*. Whitehouse Station, N.J., U.S.A.: Author.

153. Mercola, J. 2011. *If you eat processed meats are you risking your life?* Mercola.com. Retrieved 6/7/2011 from http://articles.mercola.com/sites/articles/archive/2011/01/22/if-you-eat-processed-meats-youre-risking-your-life.aspx

154. Merriam-Webster. 2012. *Ménière's disease*. Merriam-Webster's Medical Dictionary online. Retrieved 3/14/2012 from http://www2.merriam-webster.com/cgi-bin/mwmedsamp

155. Migliore, A., E. Bizzi, U. Massafra, A. Capuano, L.S. Martin Martin. 2006. Multiple chemical sensitivity syndrome in Sjögren's syndrome patients: casual association or related diseases? *Arch Environ Occup Health* 61(6):285-7.

156. Miller, J.W. 1999. Homocysteine and Alzheimer's disease. *Nutr Rev* 57(4):126-9.

157. Milovanović, B., L. Stojanović, N. Milićevik, K. Vasić, B. Bjelaković, M. Krotin. 2010. Cardiac autonomic dysfunction in patients with systemic lupus, rheumatoid arthritis and sudden death risk. *Srp Arh Celok Lek* 138(1-2):26-32.

158. Monaco, F., S. Fumero, A. Mondino, R. Mutani. 1979. Plasma and cerebrospinal fluid tryptophan in multiple sclerosis and degenerative diseases. *J Neurol Neurosurg Psychiatry* 42:640-641.

159. Moore, E. 2007. Connective Tissue Disorders: Collagen Disorders and Their Causes. *Suite101*. Retrieved 6/6/2011 from http://www.suite101.com/content/connective-tissue-disorders-a14546

160. Morris, M.C., D.A. Evans, J.L. Bienias, C.C. Tangney, D.A. Bennett, N. Aggarwal, J. Schneider, R.S. Wilson. 2003. Dietary fats and the risk of incident Alzheimer disease. *Arch Neurol* 60(2):194–200.

161. Mosby's Medical Dictionary. 2009. Elsevier. Retrieved 2/19/2011 from http://medical-dictionary.thefreedictionary.com

162. Moschiano. F., D. D'Amico, S. Usai, L. Grazzi, M. Di Stefano, E. Ciusani, N. Erba, G. Bussone. 2008. Homocysteine plasma levels in patients with migraine with aura. *Neurol Sci* 29(Suppl. 1):S173-5.

163. MSNBC. 2011. Having a baby makes mom's body turn on itself. *MSNBC News*. Retrieved 6/7/2011 from http://www.msnbc.msn.com/id/43155988/ns/health-pregnancy/t/having-baby-makes-moms-body-turn-itself/

164. MSNBC. 2010. How much vitamin D is enough? Report sets new levels. *MSNBC News*. Retrieved 4/3/2010 from http://www.msnbc.msn.com/id/40423327/ns/health-diabetes/

165. MSNBC. 2007. Excessive protein may be why some turn red. *MSNBC News*. Retrieved 1/16/2011 from http://www.msnbc.msn.com/id/20134385

166. Myhill, S. 2007a. Lack of stomach acid-hypochlorhydria-can cause lots of problems. *ProHealth*. Retrieved 4/25/2011 from http://www.prohealth.com/library/showarticle.cfm?libid=13388

167. Myhill, S. 2007b. Human Growth Hormone. Doctor Myhill.co.uk. Retrieved 3/14/2012 from http://www.drmyhill.co.uk/wiki/Human_Growth_Hormone_%28HGH%29#References

168. Myhill, S., N.E. Booth, J. McLaren-Howard. 2009. Chronic fatigue syndrome and mitochondrial dysfunction. *Int J Clin Exp Med* 2(1):1-16.

169. Nachman, R.L., S. Rafii. 2008. Platelets, petechiae, and preservation of the vascular wall. N Engl J Med 359(25):2727-8.

170. Nagy, G., A. Koncz, T. Telarico, D. Fernandez, B. Ersek, E. Buzás, A. Perl. 2010. Central role of nitric oxide in the pathogenesis of rheumatoid arthritis and systemic lupus erythematosus. *Arthritis Res Ther* 12(3):210.

171. Nakamura, Y., H. Yasuoka, M. Tsuijmoto, K. Yoshidome, M. Nakamura, K. Kakudo. 2006a. Nitric oxide in breast cancer: induction of vascular endothelial growth factor-C and correlation with metastasis and poor prognosis. *Clin Cancer Res* 12(4):1201-7.

172. Nakamura, Y., H. Yasuoka, H. Zuo, Y. Takamura, A. Miyauchi, M. Nakamura, K. Kakudo. 2006b. Nitric Oxide in Papillary Thyroid Carcinoma: Induction of Vascular Endothelial Growth Factor D and Correlation with Lymph Node Metastasis. *J Clin Endocr Metab* 91(4):1582-5.

173. National Institute of Allergy and Infectious Diseases. 2011. *Myasthenia Gravis*. Retrieved 2/18/2011 from http://www.ncbi.nlm.nih.gov/medlineplus/myastheniagravis.html

174. National Institute of Allergy and Infectious Diseases. 2010. *Food Allergy: An Overview*. Retrieved 2/13/2011 from http://www.niaid.nih.gov/topics/foodAllergy/Documents/foodallergy.pdf

175. National Institutes of Health. 2011. Diseases and Conditions Index: *Raynaud's*. U.S. Department of Health and Human Services. Retrieved 6/9/2011 from http://www.nhlbi.nih.gov/health/dci/Diseases/raynaud/ray_causes.html

176. National Institutes of Health. 2010. *Vitamin B12*. U.S. Department of Health and Human Services. Retrieved 4/3/11 from http://ods.od.nih.gov/factsheets/vitaminb12/

177. National Institutes of Health. 2009a. *Subacute combined degeneration*. U.S. Department of Health and Human Services. Retrieved 2/11/2011 from http://www.nlm.nih.gov/medlineplus/ency/article/000723.htm

178. National Institutes of Health. 2009b. *Dietary Supplement Fact Sheet: Magnesium*. U.S. Department of Health and Human Services. Retrieved 5/9/2011 from http://ods.od.nih.gov/factsheets/magnesium/

179. National Institutes of Health. 2009c. *Low Levels of Vitamin B12 May Increase Risk for Neural Tube Defects*. U.S. Department of Health and Human Services. Retrieved 6/7/2011 from http://www.nih.gov/news/health/mar2009/nichd-02.htm

180. National Institutes of Health. 2008. *Porphyria*. U.S. Department of Health and Human Services. Retrieved 3/13/2012 from http://digestive.niddk.nih.gov/ddiseases/pubs/porphyria/

181. National Institutes of Health. 2003. *Complex Regional Pain Syndrome Fact Sheet*. U.S. Department of Health and Human Services. Retrieved 3/13/2012 from http://www.ninds.nih.gov/disorders/reflex_sympathetic_dystrophy/detail_reflex_sympathetic_dystrophy.htm

182. National Institutes of Health. 2002. *Women with Endometriosis have Higher Rates of Some Diseases*. U.S. Department of Health and Human Services. Retrieved 3/4/2012 from http://www.nih.gov/news/pr/sep2002/nichd-26.htm

183. National Institutes of Health Clinical Center. 2010. *Evaluation of the Role of the Autonomic Nervous System in Sjörgren's Syndrome*. National Institute of Dental and Craniofacial Research – Clinical Trial (In Progress). Retrieved 2/19/11 from Http://clinicaltrials.gov/ct2/show/NCT00565526

184. National Jewish Health. 2010. Insulin peptide may point to a solution for type 1 diabetes. *ScienceDaily*. Retrieved 4/25/2011, from http://www.sciencedaily.com/releases/2010/06/100616133329.htm

185. Ness-Abramof, R., D.A. Nabriski, L.E. Braveman, L. Shilo, E. Weiss, T. Rashef, M.S. Shapiro, L. Shenkman. 2006. Prevalence and evaluation of B12 deficiency in patients with autoimmune thyroid disease. *Am J Med Sci* 332(3):113-22.

186. Neuman, M., P. Angulo, I. Malkiewicz, R. Jorgensen, N. Shear, E.R. Dickson, J. Haber, G. Katz, K. Lindor. 2002. Tumor Necrosis Factor-Alpha and Transforming Growth Factor-Beta Reflect Severity of Liver Damage in Primary Biliary Cirrhosis. *J Gastroenterol Hepatol* 17(2):196-202.

187. Newton, D.J., G. Kennedy, K.K.F. Chan, C.C. Lang, J.J.F. Belch, F. Khan. 2011. Large and small artery endothelial dysfunction in chronic fatigue syndrome. *Int J Cardiol* (Letter to the Editor).

188. Newton, J.L., A. Davidson, S. Kerr, N. Bhala, J. Pairman, J. Burt, D.E. Jones. 2007a. Autonomic Dysfunction in Primary Biliary Cirrhosis Correlates With Fatigue Severity. *Eur J Gastroenterol Hepatol* 19(2):125-32.

189. Newton, J.L., O. Okonkwo, K. Sutcliffe, A. Seth, J. Shin, D.E.J. Jones. 2007b. Symptoms of autonomic dysfunction in chronic fatigue syndrome. *QJM* 100(8):519-26.

190. News-Medical. 2011. Patients with rheumatoid arthritis two times more likely to have concurrent COPD. *News-Medical.Net*. Retrieved 6/6/2011 from http://www.news-medical.net/news/20110526/Patients-with-rheumatoid-arthritis-two-times-more-likely-to-have-concurrent-COPD.aspx

191. Niblett, S.H., K.E. King, R.H. Dunstan, P. Clifton-Bligh, L.A. Hoskin, T.K. Roberts, G.R. Fulcher, N.R. McGregor, J.C. Dunsmore, H.L. Butt, I. Klienbeg, T.B. Rothkirch. 2007. Hematologic and Urinary Excretion Anomalies in Patients with Chronic Fatigue Syndrome. *Exp Biol Med* 232(8):1041-9.

192. Nielsen, N.M., T. Westergaard, M. Frisch, K. Rostgaard, J. Wohlfahrt, N. Koch-Henriksen, M. Melbye, H. Hialgrim. 2006. Type 1 diabetes and multiple sclerosis: A Danish population-based cohort study. *Arch Neurol* 63(7):1001-4.

193. Nishimori, I., M. Morita, J. Kino, M. Onodera, Y. Nakazawa, K. Okazaki, Y. Yamomoto, Y. Yamamoto. 1995. Pancreatic Involvement in Patients with Sjögren's Syndrome and Primary Biliary Cirrhosis. *Int J Pancreatol* 17(1):47-54.

194. Nishimura, N., H. Okamoto, M. Yasui, K. Maeda, K. Ogura. 1959. Intermediary Metabolism of Phenylalanine and Tyrosine in Diffuse Collagen Diseases. *AMA Arch Dermatol* 80(4):466-77.

195. Nöthlings, U., L.R. Wilkens, S.P. Murhpy, J.H. Hankin, B.E. Henderson, L.N. Kolonel. Meat and Fat Intake as Risk Factors for Pancreatic Cancer: The Multiethnic Cohort Study. *J Natl Cancer Ins* 97(19):1458.

196. Oelgoetz, A.W., P.A. Oelgoetz, J. Wittenkind. 1935. The treatment of food allergy and indigestion of pancreatic origin with pancreatic enzymes. *Am J Dig Dis Nutr* 2:422-6.

197. Ohio State University. 2010. New way to study how enzymes repair DNA damage. *ScienceDaily*. Retrieved 6/7/2011, from http://www.sciencedaily.com /releases/2010/01/100128165129.htm

198. Ouzzif, Z., K. Oumghar, K. Sbai, A. Mounach, M. El Derouiche, A. El Maghraoui. 2012. Relation of plasma total homocysteine, folate and vitamin B12 levels to bone mineral density in Moroccan healthy postmenopausal women. *Rheumatol Int* 32(1):123-8.

199. Pak, K.J., S.L. Chan, M.P. Matson, 2003. Homocysteine and folate deficiency sensitize oligodendrocytes to the cell death-promoting effects of a presenilin-1 mutation and amyloid beta-peptide. Neuromolecular Med. 3(2):119-28. Pal, B., C. Gibson, J. Passmore, I.D. Griggiths, W.C. Dick. 1989. A study of headaches and migraine in Sjögren's syndrome and other rheumatic disorders. *Ann Rheum Dis* 48(4):312-6.

200. Pall, M.L. 2002. Levels of the nitric oxide synthase product citrulline are elevated in sera of chronic fatigue syndrome patients. *J Chro Fatigue Synd* 10(3/4):37-41.

201. Palm, R., G. Hallmans. 1982. Zinc and copper in multiple sclerosis. *J Neurol Neurosurg Psychiatry* 45(8):691-8.

202. Paradisi, G., H.O. Steinberg, A. Hempfling, J. Cronin, G. Hook, M.K. Shepard, A.D. Baron. 2001. Polycystic Ovary Syndrome is Associated With Endothelial Dysfunction. *Circulation* 103(10):1410-5.

203. Patarca, R., N.G. Kilmas, S. Lugtendorf, M. Antoni, M.A. Fletcher. 1994. Dysregulated expression of tumor necrosis factor in chronic fatigue syndrome: interrelations with cellular sources and patterns of soluble immune mediator expression. *Clin Infect Dis* 18(Suppl.1):S147-53.

204. Patil, N.S., A. Pashine, M.P. Belmares, W. Liu, B. Kaneshiro, J. Rabinowitz, H. McConnell, E.D. Mellins. 2001. Rheumatoid Arthritis (RA)-Associated HLA-DR Alleles Form Less Stable Complexes with Class II-Associated Invariant Chain Peptide Than Non-RA-Associated HLA-DR Alleles. *J Immunol* 167:7157-68.

205. Pearson, M. 2011. Big Money Business. Fibromyalgia Support Group Forum. Retrieved 2/20/11 from http://www.dailystrenght.org/c/Fibromyalgia

206. Pellegrino, M.J., D. Van Fossen, C. Gordon, J.M. Ryan, G.W. Waylonis. 1989. Prevalence of mitral valve prolapse in primary fibromyalgia: a pilot investigation. *Arch Phys Med Rehabil* 70(7):541-3.

207. Peterson, M. 2008. *Our Daily Meds*. Farrar, Straus and Giroux: New York, New York.

208. Petri, M., R. Roubenoff, M.R. Nadeau, J. Selhub, I.H. Rosenberg. 1996. Plasma homocysteine as a risk factor for atherothrombotic events in systemic lupus erythematosus. *Lancet* 348:1120-4.

209. Pham, C.T.N. 2008. Neutrophile serine proteases fine-tune the inflammatory response. *Int J Biochem Cell Biol* 40(6-7):1317-33

210. Phelps, J.E. 2005. *Chronic Fatigue, Fluoride & Heavy Metals*. Elektralife.com. Retrieved 2/18/2011 from http://elektralife.com/index.php?option=com_content&view=article&id=85&Itemid=92

211. Plengvidhya, V., F. Breidt Jr., Z. Lu, H.P. Fleming. 2007. DNA fingerprinting of lactic acid bacteria in sauerkraut fermentations. *Appl Environ Mircrobiol* 73(23):7697-702.

212. Pitcher, D., R. Grahame. 1982. Mitral valve prolapse and joint hypermobility: evidence for a systemic connective tissue abnormality? *Ann Rheum Dis* 41(4):352-4.

213. Polanki, P. 2004. Veggies run risk of strokes for lack of vit. B-12. *The Times of India*. Retrieved 6/6/2011 from http://articles.timesofindia.indiatimes.com/2004-07-16/pune/27157353_1_vitamin-b12-deficiency-strokes

214. Puntambekar, P., M.M. Basha, I.T. Zak, R. Madhavan. 2009. Rare sensory and autonomic disturbances associated with vitamin B12 deficiency. *J Neurol Sci* 15:287(1-2):285-7.

215. Rafalowska, J., D. Dziewulska. 1996. White Matter Injury in Amyotrophic Lateral Sclerosis (ALS). *Folia Neuropathol* 34(2):87-91.

216. Raloff, J. 1989. Dioxin: Paper's Trace. *Science News* 135(7):104.

217. Raterman, H.G., V.P. van Halm, A.E. Voskuyl, S. Simsek, B.A. Dijkmans, M.T. Nurohamed. 2008. Rheumatoid arthritis is associated with a high prevalence of hypothyroidism that amplifies its cardiovascular risk. *Ann Rheum Dis* 67(2):229-32.

218. Reed Business Information Ltd. 2006. Six years of fast-food supersizes monkeys. *NewScientist* (2556):21. Retrieved 5/24/2011 from http://www.newscientist.com/article/mg19025565.000-six-years-of-fastfood-fats-supersizes-monkeys.html

219. Regenold, W.T., P. Phatak, M.J. Makley, R.D. Stone, M.A. Kling. 2008. Cerebrospinal fluid evidence of increased extra-mitochondrial glucose metabolism implicates mitochondrial dysfunction in multiple sclerosis disease progression. *J Neurol Sci* 275(1-2):106-12.

220. Regland, B., M. Andersson, L. Abrahamsson, J. Bagby, L.E. Dyrehag, C.G. Gottfries. 1997. Increased concentrations of homocysteine in the cerebrospinal fluid in patients with fibroyalgia and chronic fatigue syndrome. *Scand J Rheumatol* 26(4):301-7.

221. Reid, M.B., Y.P. Li. 2001. Tumor necrosis factor-and muscle wasting: a cellular perspective. *Respir Res* 2(5):269-72.

222. Reyes Del Paso, G.A., S. Garrido, A. Pulgar, S. Duscheck. 2011. Autonomic cardiovascular control and responses to experimental pain stimulation in fibromyalgia syndrome. *J Psychosom Res* 70(2):125-34.

223. Reynolds, E.H., T. Bottiglieri, M. Laundy, J. Stern, J. Payan, J. Linnell, J. Faludy 1993. Subacute combined degeneration with high serum vitamin B12 level and abnormal vitamin B12 binding protein. New cause of an old syndrome. *Arch Neurol* 50(7):739-42.

224. Reynolds, E.H., T. Bottiglieri, M. Laundy, R.F. Crellin, S.G. Kirker. 1992. Vitamin B12 metabolism in multiple sclerosis. *Arch Neurol* 49(6):649-52.

225. Reynolds, E.H., J.C. Linnell, J.E. Faludy. 1991. Multiple sclerosis associated with vitamin B12 deficiency. *Arch Neurol* 48(8):808-11.

226. Roan, S. 2011. Trans fats and saturated fats could contribute to depression. *Sydney Morning Hearld*. Retrieved 5/23/2011 from http://www.smh.com.au/lifestyle/wellbeing/food-with-bad-fats-linked-to-depression-study-finds-20110127-1a6vy.html

227. Roblin, X., E. Germain, J.M. Phelip, V. Ducros, J. Pofelski, F. Heluwaert, P. Oltean, J.L. Faucheron, B. Bonaz. 2006. [Factors associated with hyperhomocysteinemia in inflammatory bowel disease: prospective study in 81 patients]. *Rev Med Interne* 27(2):106-10.

228. Rochtchina, E., J.J. Wang, V.M. Flood, P. Mitchell. 2007. Elevated serum homocysteine, low serum vitamin B12, folate, and age-related macular degeneration: the Blue Mountains Eye Study. *Am J Ophthalmol* 143(2):344-6.

229. Romagnuolo, J., R.N. Fedorak, V.C. Dias, F. Bamforth, M. Teltscher. 2001. Hyperhomocysteinemia and inflammatory bowel disease: prevalence and predictors in a cross-sectional study. *Am J Gasroenterol* 96(7):2143-9.

230. Roubenoff, R., P. Dellaripa, M.R. Nadeau, L.W. Abad, B.A. Muldoon, J. Selhub, I.H. Rosenberg. 1997. Abnormal homocysteine metabolism in rheumatoid arthritis. *Arthritis Rheum* 40(4):718-22.

231. Sandyk, R., G.I. Awerbuch. 1993 Vitamin B12 and its relationship to age of onset of multiple sclerosis. *Int J Neurosci* 71(1-4):93-9.

232. Sant, G.R., D. Kempuraj, J.E. Marchand, T.C. Theoharides. 2007. The mast cell in interstitial cystitis: role in pathophysiology and pathogenesis. *Urology* 69(4 Suppl):34-40.

233. Scaramella, J.G. 2003. Hyperhomocysteinemia and Left Internal Jugular Vein Thrombosis With Ménière's Symptom Complex. *Ear Nose Throat J* 82(11):856, 859-60, 865.

234. Schattschneider, J., K. Hartung, M. Stengel, J. Ludwig, A. Binder, G. Wasner, R. Baron. 2006. Endothelial Dysfunction in Cold Type Complex Regional Pain Syndrome. *Neurology* 67(4):673-5.

235. Seemungal, T.A., J.C. Lun, G. Davis, C. Neblett, N. Chinyepi, C. Dookhan, S. Drakes, E. Mandeville, F. Nana, S. Sethake, C.P. King, L. PintoPereira, J. Delisle, T.M. Wilkenson, J.A. Wedzicha. 2007. Plasma homocysteine is elevated in COPD patients and is related to COPD severity. *Int J Chron Obstruct Pulmon Dis* 2(3):313-21.

236. Segal, R., Y. Baumoehl, O. Elkayam, D. Levartovsky, I. Litinsky, D. Paran, I. Wigler, B. Habot, A. Leibovitz, B.A. Sela, D. Caspi. 2004. Anemia, serum vitamin B12, and folic acid in patients with rheumatoid arthritis, psoriatic arthritis, and systemic lupus erythematosus. *Rheumatol Int.* 24(1):14-9. Sendur, O.F., Y. Turan, E. Tastaban, C. Yenisey, M. Serter. 2009. Serum antioxidants and nitric oxide levels in fibromyalgia: a controlled study. *Rheumatol Int* 29(6):629-33.

237. Senol, M.G., G. Sonmez, F. Ozdag, M. Saracoglu. 2008. Reversible myelopathy with vitamin B12 deficiency. *Singapore Med J* 49(11):e330-2.

238. Seppa, N. 2000. Enzyme Shortage May Lead to Lupus. *Science News*. Retrieved 1/12/2011 from http://findarticles.com/p/articles/mi_m1200/is_24_157/ai_63323324/

239. Shemesh, Z., J. Attias, M. Ornan, N. Shapira, A. Shahar. 1993. Vitamin B12 Deficiency in Patients with Chronic-Tinnitus and Noise-Induced Hearing Loss. *Am J Otolaryng* 14(2):94-9.

240. Sieverling, C. 2002. Paul Cheney, M.D., on SSRIs and stimulants for chronic fatigue syndrome: frying the brain? *ProHealth*: June 5, 2002. Retrieved 4/25/2011 from http://www.prohealth.com/library/showarticle.cfm?libid=8480

241. Singh, A.P. 2010. *Myasthenia Gravis*. BoneandSpine.com. Retrieved 6/9/2011 from http://boneandspine.com/non-traumatic-disorders/myasthenia-gravis/

242. Soinio, M., J. Marniemi, M. Laakso, S. Lehto, T. Rönnemaa. 2004. Elevated Plasma Homocysteine Level Is an Independent Predictor of Coronary Heart Disease Events in Patients with Type 2 Diabetes Mellitus. *Ann Intern Med* 140(2):94-100.

243. Stachowiak, J. 2008. *Vitamin B12 and multiple sclerosis: people with MS may have low levels of vitamin B12*. About.com. Retrieved 4/25/2011 from http://ms.about.com/od/livingwellwithms/a/vitamin_b12.htm

244. Stampfer, M.J., M.R. Malinow, W.C. Willett, L.M. Newcomer, B. Upson, D. Ullmann, P.V. Tishler, C.H. Hennekens. 1992. A prospective study of plasma homocyst(e)ine and risk of myocardial infarction in US physicians. *J Amer Med Assoc* 268(7):877-81.

245. Steinhoff, M., U. Neisius, A. Ikoma, M. Fartasch, G. Heyer, P.S. Skov, T.A. Luger, M. Schmelz. 2003. Proteinase-Activated Receptor-2 Mediates Itch: A Novel Pathway for Pruritus in Human Skin. *J Neurosci* 23(15):6176-80.

246. Stelmasiak, Z., J. Solski, B. Jakubowska. 1995. Magnesium concentration in plasma and erythrocytes in MS. *Acta Neurol Scan* 92(1):109-11.

247. Stitt, P., M. Knickelbine, S. Knickelbine. 1980. *Fighting the food giants*. Natural Press: Manitowoc, WI.

248. StopTransFats.com. 2007. *Danger of Trans Fats--In Distorting Cell Membranes and Cell Structures*. Retrieved 6/7/2011 from http://www.stop-trans-fat.com/danger-of-trans-fats.html

249. Suryanarayan, D. 2010. Veggie Indians more prone to heart disease. *Daily News & Anaysis*. Retrieved 6/6/2011 from http://www.dnaindia.com/mumbai/report_veggie-indians-more-prone-to-heart-disease_1443372

250. Swadzba, J., T. Iwaniec, J. Musial. 2011. Increased level of tumor necrosis factor-a in patients with antiphospholipid syndrome: marker not only of inflammation but also of the prothrombotic state. *Rheumatol Int* 31(3):307-13.

251. Tangney, C.C., N.T. Aggarwal, H. Li, R.S. Wilson, C. Decarli, D.A. Evans, M.C. Morris. 2011. Vitamin B12, cognition, and brain MRI measures: a cross-sectional examination. *Neurology* 77(13):1276-82.

252. Taylor, D.A. 2004. Funky Chicken: Consumes Exposed to Arsenic in Poultry. *Environ Health Persp* 112(1):A50.

253. Teicholz, N. 2004. Heart Breaker. *Gourmet* June:103.

254. Tekin, G., A. Tekin, E.B. Kiliçarslan, B. Haydardedeoğlu, T. Katircibaşi, T. Koçum, T. Erol, Y. Cölkesen, A.T. Sezgin, H. Müderrisoğlu. 2008. Altered Autonomic Neural Control of the Cardiovascular System in Patients With Polycystic Ovary Syndrome. *Int J Cardiol* 130(1):49-55.

255. Tektonidou, M.G., N. Varsou, G. Kotoulas, A. Antoniou, H.M. Moutsopoulos. 2006. Cognitive Deficits in Patients With Antiphospholipid Syndrome. *Arch Intern Med* 166:2278-84.

256. Tewthanom, K., S. Janwityanuchit, K. Totemchockchyakarn, D. Panomvana. 2008. Correlation of lipid peroxidation and glutathione levels with severity of systemic lupus erythematosus: a pilot study from single center. *J Pharm Pharm Sci* 11(3):30-4.

257. tfX.org. 2004. *Trans fats and health—quotes*. The Campaign Against Trans Fats in Food. Retrieved 6/7/2011 from http://www.tfx.org.uk/page31.html

258. The American Heritage Science Dictionary. 2005. Houghton Mifflin Company, Internet. Retrieved 2/19/11 from www.thefreedictionary.com/

259. Thornalley, P.J., R. Babaei-Jadidi, H. Al Ali, N. Rabbani, A. Antonysunil, J. Larkin, A. Ahmed, G. Rayman, C.W. Bodmer. 2007. High prevalence of low plasma thiamine concentration in diabetes linked to a marker of vascular disease. *Diabetologia* 50(10):2164-70.

260. Tishler, M., T. Smorodin, M. Vazina-Amit, Y. Ramot, M. Koffler, B. Fishel. 2003. Fibromyalgia in diabetes mellitus. Rheumatol Int 23(4):171-3.

261. Toussirot, E., M. Bahjaoui-Bouhaddi, J. Poncet, S. Cappelle, M. Henriet, D. Wending, J. Regnard. 1999. Abnormal Autonomic Cardiovascular Control in Ankylosing Spondylitis. *Ann Rheum Dis* 58(8):481-7.

262. Triantafyllou, N., M.E. Evangelopoulos, V.K. Kimiskidis, E. Kararizou, F. Boufidou, K.N. Fountoulakis, M. Siamouli, C. Nikolaou, C. Sfagos, N. Vlaikidis, D. Vassilopoulos. 2008. Increased plasma homocysteine levels in patients with multiple sclerosis and depression. *Ann Gen Psychiatry* 7:17.

263. Troen, A.M., M. Shea-Budgell, B. Shukitt-Hale, D.E. Smith, J. Selhub, I.H. Rosenberg. 2008. B-vitamin deficiency causes hyperhomocysteinemia and vascular cognitive impairment in mice. *P Natl Acad Sci* 105(34):12474.

264. Uemura, T., M. Itoh, N. Kikuchi. 1980. Autonomic Dysfunction On the Affected Side in Ménière's Disease. *Acta Otolaryngol* 89(1-2):109-17.

265. University of California – San Francisco. 2006. Autoimmune Disease Triggered If T Cellls Miss A Single Protein Early On. *ScienceDaily*. Retrieved 2/18/2011 from http://www.sciencedaily.com/releases/2006/11/061121232053.htm

266. University of Chicago. 2010. *Types of Peripheral Neuropathy—Systemic/Metabolic*. Center for Peripheral Neuropathy. Retrieved 3/4/2012 from http://peripheralneuropathycenter.uchicago.edu/learnaboutpn/typesofpn/systemic/nutrition.shtml

267. University of Gothenburg. 2010. New findings on autoimmune diseases. *ScienceDaily*. Retrieved 211/2011, from http://www.sciencedaily.com/releases/2010/10/101010183705.htm

268. University of Illinois at Chicago. 2011. Reduced levels of an important neurotransmitter found in multiple sclerosis patients. *ScienceDaily*. Retrieved April 3, 2011, from http://www.sciencedaily.com/releases/2011/02/110211124623.htm

269. University of Michigan Health System. 2003. High Heart Disease Risk For Lupus Patients May Be Linked To Rapid Death Of Blood Vessel Lining Cells. *ScienceDaily*. Retrieved 2/12 2011 from http://www.sciencedaily.com/releases/2003/11/031113070845.htm

270. U.S. Department of Agriculture. 2002. Homocysteine: The New "Bad Boy" of Vascular Disease. Retrieved 4/2/2012 from http://www.ars.usda.gov/is/AR/archive/may02/vasc0502.htm

271. U.S. Dept of Health and Human Services. 2011. *How to Understand and Use the Nutrition Facts Label*. U.S. Food and Drug Administration. Retrieved 5/23/2011 from http://www.fda.gov/food/labelingnutrition/consumerinformation/ucm078889.htm

272. U.S. Dept of Health and Human Services. 2003. *Trans Fat Press Conference*. U.S. Food and Drug Administration. Retrieved 5/24/2011 from http://www.hhs.gov/news/speech/2003/030709.html

273. U.S. Food and Drug Administration. 2006. *Total Diet Study: Market Baskets* 1991-3 through 2003-4. Retrieved 2/11/2011 from http://www.fda.gov/downloads/Food/FoodSafety/FoodContaminantsAdulteration/TotalDietStudy/UCM184304.pdf

274. van Meurs, J.B., R.A. Dhonukshe-Rutten, S.M. Pluijm, K. van der Klift, R. de Jonge, J. Lindemans, L.C. de Groot, A. Hofman, J.C. Witteman, J.P. van Leeuwen, M.M. Breteler, P. Lips, H.A. Pols, A.G. Uitterlinden. 2004. Homocysteine levels and the risk of osteoporotic fracture. *New Engl J Med* 350(20):233-41.

275. van Staa, T.P., P. Geusens, J.W. Bijlsma, H.G. Leufkens, C. Cooper. 2006. Clinical assessment of the long-term risk of fracture in patients with rheumatoid arthritis. *Arthritis Rheum* 54(10):3104-12.

276. Varghese, M., W. Zhao, J. Wang, A. Cheng, X. Qian, A. Chaudhry, L. Ho, G.M. Pasinetti. 2011. Mitochondrial bioenergetics is defective in presymptomatic Tg2576 AD Mice. *Transl Neurosci* 2011:2(1):1-2.

277. Vasan, R.S., A. Beiser, R.B. D'Agostino, D. Levy, J. Selhub, P.F. Jaques, I.H. Rosenberg, P.W.F. Wilson. 2003. Plasma Homocysteine and Risk for Congestive Heart Failure in Adults Without Prior Myocardial Infarction. *J Amer Med Assoc* 289(10):1251-7.

278. Velicer, C.M., S.R. Heckbert, J.W. Lampe, J.D. Potter, C.A. Robertson, S.H. Taplin. 2004. Antibiotic Use in Relation to the Risk of Breast Cancer. *J Amer Med Assoc* 291(7):827-35.

279. Vogiatzoglou, A., H. Refsum, C. Johnston, S.M. Smith, K.M. Bradley, C. de Jager, M.M. Budge, A.D. Smith. 2008. Vitamin B12 status and rate of brain volume loss in community-dwelling elderly. *Neurology* 71(11):826-32.

280. Vollset, S.E., H. Refsum, L.M. Irgens, B.M. Emblem, A. Tverdal, H.K. Gjessing, A.L.B. Monsen, P.M. Ueland. 2000. Plasma total homocysteine, pregnancy complications, and adverse pregnancy outcomes: the Hordaland Homocysteine Study. *Am J Clin Nutr* 70(4):962-8.

281. Walport, M.J. 2000. Lupus, DNase and defective disposal of cellular debris. *Nat Genet* 25:135-6.

282. Wanchu, A., M. Khullar, A. Sud, P. Bambery. 2000. Elevated nitric oxide production in patients with Sjögren's syndrome. *Clin Rheumatol* 19(5):360-4.

283. WebMD. 2011. *Rheumatoid Arthritis Skin Problems*. WebMD.com. Retrieved 6/9/2011 from http://www.webmd.com/rheumatoid-arthritis/rheumatoid-arthritis-skin-problems

284. Wegelius, O., F. Fyhrquist, P.L. Adner. 1987. Sjögren's Syndrome Associated with Vitamin B12 Deficiency. *Scan Jnl Rheumatol* 16(1):184-190.

285. Wellness.com. 2011. *Vitamin B12.* Wellness.com Inc. Retrieved 4/26/2011 from http://www.wellness.com/reference/vitamins/vitamin-b12/dosing-and-safety

286. Wells, L.J. *Poor stomach acid output can lead to serious disorders.* Wellspring Integrated Healthcare. Retrieved 4/3/11 from http://drlyndawells.com/PoorStomachAcid.aspx

287. Whitaker, H. 2007. *Chronic Fatigue Syndrome and Hyperthyroidism are an "Official Couple."* EzineArticles.com. Retrieved 6/9/2011 from http://ezinearticles.com/?Chronic-Fatigue-Syndrome-and-Hypothyroidism-are-an-Official-Couple&id=743241

288. Whitaker, H. 2006. *The Cost of Record Heat Hits More Than Just Your Wallet.* PRWeb. Retrieved 1/21/11 from http://www.prweb.com/releases/2006/07/prweb415458.htm

289. Wikipedia. 2011a. *Homocysteine.* Retrieved 6/6/2011 from http://en.wikipedia.org/wiki/Homocysteine#cite_note-NEJM2006a-12

290. Wikipedia. 2011b. *Dysautonomia.* Retrieved 2/20/2011 from http://en.wikipedia.org/wiki/Dysautonomia#cite_note-8

291. Wiley-Blackwell. 2010. Heart attack risk increases rapidly after rheumatoid arthritis is diagnosed. *ScienceDaily.* Retrieved 5/8/2011 from http://www.sciencedaily.com/releases/2010/12/101206093216.htm

292. Williams, R.M. 1999. Lupus and Environmental Risk Factors. *Townsend Letter* Aug:48-50.

293. Wu, M.Y., K.H. Chao, J.H. Yang, T.H. Lee, Y.S. Yang, H.N. Ho. 2003. Nitric oxide synthesis is increased in the endometrial tissue of women with endometriosis. *Hum Reprod* 18(12):2688-94.

294. Yajnik, C.S., S.S. Deshpande, H.G. Lubree, S.S. Naik, D.S. Bhat, B.S. Uradey, J.A. Deshpande, S.S. Rege, H. Refsum, J.S. Yudkin. 2006. Vitamin B12 Deficiency and Hyperhomocysteinemia in Rural and Urban Indians. *J Assoc Phys India* 54:775-82.

295. Yakut, M., Y. Üstün, G. Kabaçam, I. Soykan. 2010. Serum vitamin B12 and folate status in patients with inflammatory bowel diseases. *Eur J Intern Med* 21:320-3.

296. Yamada, T., M. Nishimura, H. Mita. 2007. Increased number of apoptotic endothelial cells in bladder of interstitial cystitis patients. *World J Urol* 25(4):407-13.

297. Yamasaki, K., A. Di Nardo, A. Bardan, M. Murakami, T. Ohtake, A. Coda, R.A. Dorschner, C. Bonnart, P. Descargues, A. Hovnanian, V.B. Morhenn, R.L. Gallo. 2007. Increased serine protease activity and cathelicidin promotes skin inflammation in Rosacea. *Nat Med* 13:975-80.

298. Yasui, M., Y. Yase, K. Ando, K. Adachi, M. Mukoyama, K. Ohsugi. 1990. Magnesium concentration in brains from multiple sclerosis patients. *Acta Neurol Scand* 81(3):197-200.

299. Yasutomo, K., T. Horiuchi, S. Kagami, H. Tsukamoto, C. Hashimura, M. Urushihara, Y. Kuroda. 2001. Mutation of DNASE1 in people with systemic lupus erythematosus. *Nat Genet* 28(4):313-4.

300. Yiamouyiannis, J. 1986. Fluoride: The Aging Factor. *Health Action Press*: Deleware, OH.

301. Yilmaz, A., R.A. Sari, M. Gundogdu, N. Kose, E. Dag. 2005. Trace elements and some extracellular antioxidant proteins levels in serum of patients with systemic lupus erythematosus. *Clin Rheumatol* 24(4):331-5.

302. Yunus M.B., J.W. Dailey, J.C. Aldag, A.T. Masi, P.C. Jobe. 1992. Plasma tryptophan and other amino acids in primary fibromyalgia: a controlled study. J Rheumatol. Jan;19(1):90-4. Zhang, C., Y. Cai, M.T. Adachi, S. Oshiro, T. Aso, R.J. Kaufman, S. Kitajima. 2001. Homocysteine induces programmed cell death in human vascular endothelial cells through activation of the unfolded protein response. *J Biol Chem* 276(38):35867-74.

303. Zoccolella, S., C. Bendotti, E. Beghi, G. Logroscino. 2010. Homocysteine Levels and Amyotrophic Lateral Sclerosis: A Possible Link. *Amyotroph Lateral Scler* 11(1-2):140-7.

304. Zoccolella, S., I.L. Simone, P. Lamberti, V. Samarelli, R. Tortelli, L. Serlenga, G. Logroscino. 2008. Elevated Plasma Homocysteine Levels in Patients With Amyotrophic Lateral Sclerosis. *Neurology* 70(3):222-5.

305. Zykova, S.N., A.A. Tveita, O.P. Rekvig. 2010. Renal Dnase1 Enzyme Activity and Protein Expression is Selectively Shut Down in Murine and Human Membranoproliverative Lupus Nephritis. *PlosONE* 5(8):e12096.